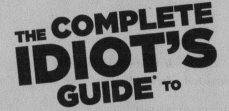

THE COMPLETE IDIOT'S GUIDE TO

Raw Food Detox

by Adam A. Graham

ALPHA
A member of Penguin Group (USA) Inc.

ALPHA BOOKS

Published by the Penguin Group

Penguin Group (USA) Inc., 375 Hudson Street, New York, New York 10014, USA

Penguin Group (Canada), 90 Eglinton Avenue East, Suite 700, Toronto, Ontario M4P 2Y3, Canada (a division of Pearson Penguin Canada Inc.)

Penguin Books Ltd., 80 Strand, London WC2R 0RL, England

Penguin Ireland, 25 St. Stephen's Green, Dublin 2, Ireland (a division of Penguin Books Ltd.)

Penguin Group (Australia), 250 Camberwell Road, Camberwell, Victoria 3124, Australia (a division of Pearson Australia Group Pty. Ltd.)

Penguin Books India Pvt. Ltd., 11 Community Centre, Panchsheel Park, New Delhi—110 017, India

Penguin Group (NZ), 67 Apollo Drive, Rosedale, North Shore, Auckland 1311, New Zealand (a division of Pearson New Zealand Ltd.)

Penguin Books (South Africa) (Pty.) Ltd., 24 Sturdee Avenue, Rosebank, Johannesburg 2196, South Africa

Penguin Books Ltd., Registered Offices: 80 Strand, London WC2R 0RL, England

International Standard Book Number: 978-1-61564-0-942
Library of Congress Catalog Card Number: 2010919335

13 12   8 7 6 5 4 3

Interpretation of the printing code: The rightmost number of the first series of numbers is the year of the book's printing; the rightmost number of the second series of numbers is the number of the book's printing. For example, a printing code of 11-1 shows that the first printing occurred in 2011.

Printed in the United States of America

Note: This publication contains the opinions and ideas of its author. It is intended to provide helpful and informative material on the subject matter covered. It is sold with the understanding that the author and publisher are not engaged in rendering professional services in the book. If the reader requires personal assistance or advice, a competent professional should be consulted.

The author and publisher specifically disclaim any responsibility for any liability, loss, or risk, personal or otherwise, which is incurred as a consequence, directly or indirectly, of the use and application of any of the contents of this book.

Most Alpha books are available at special quantity discounts for bulk purchases for sales promotions, premiums, fund-raising, or educational use. Special books, or book excerpts, can also be created to fit specific needs.

For details, write: Special Markets, Alpha Books, 375 Hudson Street, New York, NY 10014.

Publisher: *Marie Butler-Knight*

Associate Publisher: *Mike Sanders*

Executive Managing Editor: *Billy Fields*

Acquisitions Editor: *Tom Stevens*

Development Editor: *Jennifer Bowles*

Senior Production Editor: *Janette Lynn*

Copy Editor: *Lisanne Jensen*

Cover Designer: *Kurt Owens*

Book Designers: *William Thomas, Rebecca Batchelor*

Indexer: *Brad Herriman*

Layout: *Brian Massey*

Proofreader: *John Etchison*

Dedicated to BJA.

Contents

10   Raw Spreads, Sauces, and Dressings 123

11   Raw Soups and Salads 139

Appendixes

Introduction

You may have heard a lot about the benefits of eating raw foods in general—and the idea of following a raw food detoxification program specifically—but are hesitant to jump in head first without a bit more information. Well, you've definitely come to the right place to learn how raw food detox can dramatically alter the direction of your health and life.

From losing weight to waking up with clearer skin, raw food detox has the capability to enhance your body while eliminating dangerous toxins that we are subjected to in our food, homes, and just about everywhere.

Learning the basics is important, and that's where we'll start. You'll determine your recommended level of raw food intensity as you begin and learn to prepare a multitude of delicious and easy-to-make recipes. You'll also find out about foods that are vital for healing as well as activities you can do to help the detox process along.

How This Book Is Organized

There are five parts to this book:

Part 1, The Raw Essentials, provides you with the basics on raw food detox and why it works to create vitality and health, as well as an overview of the type of toxins we encounter every day and how we can help our bodies through the detoxification process.

Part 2, Getting Started, will help you determine which program—A, B, C, or D—is best for you and what each 15-day menu looks like, as well as make recommendations on preparing your kitchen and your life for the detox adventure.

Part 3, Recipes for Success, consists of all the recipes you will need, from snacks to soups to juices, to successfully embark on the raw food detox program.

Part 4, Let Raw Food Be Thy Medicine, discusses the potent nutrition available to your body when you follow the raw food detox plan and explains a number of unusual healing and superfoods that can help you on your way.

Part 5, The Newly Detoxed You, will provide you with tips on how to maintain your success and apply detoxification to your home and environment to promote a healthy atmosphere.

Helpful Notes

You'll come across many helpful notes throughout the book that will provide you with some additional information. Watch for these:

> **DEFINITIONS**
>
> Here, you'll find explanations of raw food terminology and some other health-related jargon.

> **RAWESOME TIPS**
>
> These will provide you with advice and hints on a variety of raw food detox topics.

> **DETOXER'S ALERT**
>
> Be sure to check out these specific health warnings and alerts.

> **FRESH FACTS**
>
> These contain a wealth of interesting facts, figures, and amusing trivia for your reading pleasure.

Acknowledgments

Family and friends are at the heart of all great endeavors and this project is no exception. I am blessed to have the support of my parents and two brothers throughout my lifetime of projects and adventures. A heart-to-heart hug and thank you goes out to one of my biggest supporters and motivators, Leah Hudson.

Much of my inspiration came from my local raw food community at Friday Soup Nights and JaxRaw potlucks. I thank all of you for your tasty creativity and support. The opportunity to share the message of raw food detox came as a result of a number of synchronicities. It all started with a friend request on Facebook by Kelly Jad'on, which led to a connection with chef and author Mark Reinfeld, and eventually publishing agent Marilyn Allen.

Thanks spread out from those beginnings like a pebble in a pond to writer and chef Elizabeth Scott and editor Tom Stevens. A final thank you goes out to the ever-expanding raw food–conscious individuals and groups around the world who are my mentors and peers that keep expanding and sharing the message of a healthy and sustainable way of life. We are blessed. Keep it Live!

Special Thanks to the Technical Reviewer

The Complete Idiot's Guide to Raw Food Detox was reviewed by an expert who double-checked the accuracy of what you'll learn here, to help us ensure that this book gives you everything you need to know about raw food detox. Special thanks are extended to Rhonda Lerner.

Trademarks

All terms mentioned in this book that are known to be or are suspected of being trademarks or service marks have been appropriately capitalized. Alpha Books and Penguin Group (USA) Inc. cannot attest to the accuracy of this information. Use of a term in this book should not be regarded as affecting the validity of any trademark or service mark.

The Raw Essentials

Before embarking on any type of program, it's essential to understand the ins and outs of what you'll be doing—and in this part, you'll do just that. From learning why detoxification is necessary to understanding the process, you'll be well equipped with information. We'll start with a brief discussion of the raw food program and explain how body detoxification works. We'll follow up with a good understanding of the plethora of toxins in our world and how they may affect your health. After a detailed discussion of how this raw food detoxification will make you the best and healthiest you can be, you'll find out about reinforcements you can call in—in the form of exercise and other practices that will serve to make your detoxification even more successful and enjoyable.

The Ins and Outs of Raw Food Detox

In This Chapter

- What raw food is all about
- Why we need detoxifying
- How raw food detox works

Welcome to the beginning of a happier and healthier you! Getting to know the basic concepts behind the raw food detox program you are about to embark upon is your first step toward vibrancy, increased energy, and a stable and healthy weight. Get ready to explore the exciting idea of raw food detoxification.

Why detox at all? And why raw food, you may ask? What exactly is meant by raw food, anyway? This chapter will shed a bright light on the subject so you can better understand why a raw food detox is the way to go.

You'll also learn about the process of detoxification that regularly occurs in your body and how some added assistance can make a world of difference in successfully ridding your body of unwanted toxins that could promote disease and early aging. Aiding your body's normal detox process will keep you as toxin-free as possible and as happy and healthy as you should be.

Raw Food Defined

Raw food and the *raw food diet* have been gaining press, popularity, and momentum in recent years. Many practitioners, along with some competitive athletes and Hollywood elite, swear by its healing properties. In reality, everyone has eaten at least a partial raw food diet whether they know it or not—it's nothing sensational or new.

It's just eating fresh, natural, uncooked whole foods. If you've ever chowed down on slabs of watermelon in the summer, eaten a bowl of fresh cherries, or enjoyed a simple green salad, you've eaten raw foods. Incidentally, I bet that watermelon made you feel refreshed and satisfied. Well that's just one benefit that raw foods and raw food detox can offer—but more on that later.

> **DEFINITION**
>
> A **raw food diet** consists of whole foods that have not been processed or heated higher than 118 degrees Fahrenheit.

The Uncooked Theory

Why opt for uncooked food? The explanation is pretty simple. Cooking can destroy the naturally occurring enzymes and nutrients in food that are beneficial to good health, prevent disease, and halt rapid aging. The more cooked foods we eat, the less likely we are to ingest these vital substances—and the more likely we are to become susceptible to illness, weight gain, and overall poor health. In particular, a raw food diet consisting primarily of plant-based foods provides us with healthy *antioxidants* and *phytonutrients* that are believed to give us an advantage in keeping us free of disease and battling the many toxins to which we are exposed. Although we are still learning about the role these very important nutrients play in human health, we certainly know that cooking often lessens the nutrients available to us, and that's a very good reason to eat as many raw foods as we can. As you will see, these vital enzymes and nutrients play an important role in the raw food detoxification you're about to enjoy.

> **DEFINITION**
>
> **Antioxidants,** which include vitamins A, C, and E, prevent free radical (unstable and harmful atoms that can be present in human tissue) damage in the body, which can lead to premature aging and disease.
>
> **Phytonutrients** are naturally occurring, plant-based chemicals that, when consumed as part of a healthy diet, are believed to help ward off disease and illness.

Raw foods also have a much higher water content than cooked foods (think of the watermelon), which assists in maintaining proper hydration in the body. This helps us absorb water-soluble vitamins, such as vitamin C and B complex vitamins that require constant replenishment as they cannot be stored, which are so plentiful in nature and ultimately keep our skin and complexions youthful and glowing.

And if that's not enough, raw, plant-based foods naturally contain a high amount of fiber, which studies have shown is essential to good digestive health and instrumental in weight control.

FRESH FACT

Cooking foods at high temperatures can destroy enzymes; reduce the amount of vitamins, minerals, protein, and fiber; and even result in the formation of free radicals and toxins.

Vegetarian or Not?

If you're wondering whether a raw food diet is necessarily a vegetarian one, the answer is, "That depends." Many raw foodists start out eating only a portion of uncooked, plant-based foods while continuing to dine on cooked fish, eggs, chicken, or even beef. Eventually, the enjoyment and benefits of eating raw entice many folks to continue on, eating a greater percentage of raw food and eventually embracing what is known as a vegan lifestyle. Vegans, through conscious choice, do not eat or use any products derived from animals. Although many raw food enthusiasts are vegan, it is not necessary to become one in order to embark on a raw food detox. You just may decide, however, that continuing to eat in such a healthy fashion might be the logical and desirable way to go.

Detox Defined

If *detoxification* sounds like pretty serious business, that's because it is. Consider the seriousness of detoxing from alcohol or drugs or from the ingestion of, say, heavy metals or poisons—all of which are very serious. What you may not realize is that this very serious business of detoxification is actually a natural and normal bodily function that goes on inside us every day. External toxins that have entered the body (and even some internal toxins made by the body) are neutralized or removed with every breath you take, in every waking moment, and even while you sleep.

DEFINITION

Detoxification is the removal or neutralizing of toxic substances in a living organism and is a naturally occurring process in the human body.

Toxins are not just ingested from the outside. If you're living, breathing, and burning calories, you're producing toxins that need to be managed. Because the human body is essentially a work in progress, it actually creates a number of toxins in the formation of new cells and through the natural aging process. These toxic by-products, along with those toxins that we ingest and breathe in, must also be removed or neutralized. Most of the time, your body does its job quite well without needing additional help. Sometimes, however, especially in this all-too-toxic world we live in, your body needs a boost.

Cleaning Your Internal House

Let's suppose your body is a house, and external toxins are the dirt you track in on the bottom of your shoes—or the vehicle exhaust that drifts in through your windows. In a clean, efficiently run household, the dirt gets swept up and disposed of without much effort. You can even help this process by trying not to track dirt inside, establishing a strict "no shoes" policy, or closing the windows. Clearly, the less dirt you track in, the less there is to sweep up—and that goes for toxins, too.

But what about internally generated toxins—all the unwanted "dirt" from natural and unnatural processes that occur inside the body? For example, let's say you spill some juice, wipe it up with a paper towel, and then throw the paper towel away. That paper towel is now waste created while cleaning up a spill. No need to panic, however. Spills like this happen inside us all the time, and the body has a "clean-up staff" that's always on call to take care of these little messes. But there's a catch.

Taking Out the Trash

Just because these toxins have been collected or put in the trash doesn't mean they've actually been removed from the body. We're often too busy to take out the trash, and the same goes for our bodies. Because the body often has its hands full taking care of vital life processes, sometimes toxins have to be swept aside instead of being immediately removed. And they can end up collecting, much like trash does in the house—in dark corners, under beds, in closets, in the basement, up in the attic, and in the garage.

The most common places where the body collects and stores toxins are the same places it tends to store fat: around the waist, hips, thighs, and buttocks. In fact, it is often in these fat cells that toxins are securely sealed away and stored. Here, they can accumulate and pose a serious health risk by playing host to numerous unwanted parasites, including yeast and mold, and by jeopardizing the functioning of our organs. If not eventually removed, toxic buildup can contribute to a host of physical ailments and some pretty serious diseases.

Simply put, detoxification is the act of taking out the trash. As long as the amount of toxins coming in (including internally generated toxins) does not exceed the body's natural ability to detox, health is, for the most part, adequately maintained. When the balance shifts in favor of toxins, however, health declines and disease begins to manifest in the body. Excess toxins in the body can contribute to accelerated aging and degenerative diseases—things we would all love to avoid.

By assisting the body in its detoxification, we can make a dramatic difference in our health and slow down or even prevent many age-related conditions. Through a combination of proper nutrition and the elimination of toxins, we can achieve dramatic results. By applying these principles in your own life, you may be able to improve and extend the life in your cells (quite specifically)—and in turn, the life in you (more generally). That's seriously good news.

FRESH FACT

In 1912, Nobel Prize winner Dr. Alexis Carrel demonstrated in his laboratory the ability to keep living cells in an embryonic chicken heart alive beyond their normal life expectancies by providing proper nutrition and removing toxins.

Who Needs It?

If detoxification implies good health, then just about anyone can benefit from a detox diet to some degree—young or elderly, active or inactive, underweight or overweight, and sick or healthy. This doesn't mean everyone should approach detoxification in the same way or degree, however. Someone who is sick will naturally need to do things differently than a competitive athlete. For some, a detox plan can be as simple as starting the day with 20 ounces of distilled water with fresh squeezed lemon juice or stopping eating at 6 P.M. For others, a more aggressive approach may be in order.

Here are some of the physical signs and problems that could indicate a detox may be beneficial for your body:

- Allergies

- Aches and pains

- Acne

- Chronic congestion

- Headaches, including migraines

- Inability to lose or gain weight

- Joint pain

- Rash or eczema

- Frequent colds

- Constipation

- Heartburn or excess gas

DETOXER'S ALERT

Always consult your healthcare provider before embarking on any detoxification program, even if for a short period of time.

The Basics of Detox

Understanding the basic process of detoxification is pretty easy. It consists of two distinct phases that are equally important in eliminating toxins from the body. As mentioned earlier, the body squirrels away toxins by imprisoning them in fat cells as well as organ tissue. There's a reason for this. You may have noticed when cleaning greasy dishes that water alone cannot dissolve fat. That's exactly the reason why the body has encased toxins in fat. For your protection, they are fat-soluble when placed into storage so they can't go wandering off in your body without close monitoring.

Unlocking the Toxins

In order for toxins to be eliminated, they first need to be released from their fatty captivity. This is what occurs during phase one: stored toxins are converted back into water-soluble chemicals that can be removed through the various elimination channels of the body, including sweat, breath, urine, and feces.

Think of your fat cells as "jail cells" for toxins. When the convicts are in their cells, they cause few problems. The liver acts as the warden, managing all things toxic in the body. But the liver can't be overworked or undernourished, or its performance might be negatively altered. Consuming foods that support the liver is a great way to prepare for detoxing the body, and this is essentially what should occur during phase one of detoxification as the toxins begin their release.

Phase two is essentially the subsequent elimination stage. If the body is drained of energy or is deficient in vital nutrients, however (which is often the case for many of us), these newly released, water-soluble toxins can wreak havoc in the body.

Escorting Them Out

Now that the cells are open, you need to escort these unruly toxins from the premises. The key to a successful phase two is arming the body with a crack security team made up of antioxidants, enzymes, and amino acids—all things we'll learn about in greater depth later on and which come primarily from the foods we eat.

Be mindful that phase two detoxification shouldn't be taken lightly. If the liver is ill-equipped to dump these toxins and the systems of elimination aren't prepared, these toxic marauders can cause serious damage. This includes all those free radicals that must be kept in check and are responsible for so much early aging and disease. In the next chapter, you'll see why raw food ingestion is key to this process. For now, know that what you consume during a detox is critical to its overall result.

RAWESOME TIP

Foods known to support liver function include garlic, onions, wheatgrass, carrots, beets, burdock, Jerusalem artichokes (sunchokes), dandelions, parsley, lemons, grapefruit, and spinach.

What About a Cleanse?

You may have heard people announce they are "doing a cleanse" or seen advertisements for all sorts of internal body cleansing products and wondered what the difference is between detoxification and cleansing. In general, cleansing and detox go hand in hand, although a "cleanse" is normally undertaken to clean out specific systems or organs of the body, such as a "colon cleanse."

Cleanses usually occur for very short periods of time (perhaps only a day or two) and often entail the ingestion of simple liquids or supplements. The intent is also to detox, but not to the extent that an actual detoxification protocol can achieve. A cleanse is also sometimes referred to as a "flush" and may target the liver or gall bladder, for example. All in all, a detoxification such as the one you'll embark on in this book is usually more serious than a cleanse and is a lot more thorough.

Bottom Line Results

Raw food detox restores health and initiates healing without negative side effects. What exactly can you expect from a raw food detoxification program, and what exciting results can you anticipate?

Health and Vitality

Have you ever met a centenarian? That's a person who has lived to or passed the age of 100. In developed modern countries such as ours, statistics regarding childhood disease sound an alarm that this generation of children may not outlive their parents. Obesity, diabetes, cancer, heart disease, arthritis, hypertension … the list continues for diseases afflicting more and more children.

In John Robbins' book *Healthy at 100*, he specifically researched the cultures and communities around the world with the highest concentration of centenarians: the Hunza Valley in Pakistan; Okinawa, Japan; Vilcabamba, Ecuador; and the Republic of Abkhazia. All these long-lived communities have some factors in common:

- They consume little to no processed foods.

- The majority of their calories are eaten raw.

- They eat live, fermented foods and unpasteurized dairy (if any).

- They consume minimal animal protein, and what they do eat is caught wild or free range.

- They maintain an active lifestyle.

Weight Control

Weight control is usually the driving force behind the desire to change one's diet. If you're trying to lose, or possibly gain, weight, raw foods and detox can help get you to your ideal weight. Minimizing processed foods and increasing raw, whole foods will make a difference in your weight. Raw food detox can balance weight by removing toxins, hydrating the body, exchanging unhealthy fats for healthy fats, providing fiber for proper elimination, providing a full spectrum of nutrients, and incorporating physical activity to build muscle and eliminate fat.

Water weight plays a major role in bringing balance to weight issues. How can a person have both water weight and be dehydrated? In cases of toxicity and an acidic pH, the body stores water within its cells to dilute toxins and buffer acids. This water is not available for hydrating the systems of the body or flushing out toxins.

One indicator of chronic dehydration is a dark-yellow urine color accompanied by a strong odor. With hydration, this color lightens and the odor becomes less pronounced. By adding a supply of pure water from fresh fruits and vegetables as well as alkalizing minerals, the body responds by dumping all the stored water in its cells. This purging may appear as a dramatic loss in weight over a short period of time. Once water weight has been eliminated, a person's weight loss may slow down or even stop. At this point, it's time to work on removing toxic fat deposits, which takes more time than purging water weight. Water weight often comes back—and quickly—when unbalanced, processed, or toxic foods are reintroduced. This is just the body protecting itself once again. By maintaining a higher percentage of healthy, hydrating raw foods in your diet, you can ward off this water weight for good.

Disease and Inflammation Prevention

Inflammation is defined as part of the biological response in the body by vascular tissue to harmful stimuli (pathogens, toxins, and irritants). This can be as simple as a bug bite. But what happens when a lot of what you put in and on your body is a toxic irritant? Inflammation at chronic levels can occur, and disease ensues.

Inflammation is the body's attempt to remove unwelcome substances before infection occurs. If it doesn't achieve this goal, it's possible that infection can occur in the weakest parts of the body. The result of chronic inflammation is cell destruction.

Another variety of inflammation has been associated with obesity: systemic inflammation. It's characterized by the presence of interleukin, part of the immune response system. During a clinical study of systemic inflammation, the problem was remedied in four weeks by initiating a low-calorie diet. Imagine the results by just eating raw foods. A majority of raw foods are capable of relieving inflammatory conditions, and there is a special category of raw foods known to be anti-inflammatory.

Highly Inflammatory Foods	Anti-Inflammatory Foods
Alcohol	Berries
Caffeine	Garlic
Corn and corn-based foods	Green, leafy vegetables
Dairy (especially cheese)	Onion
Gluten products: grains	Pineapple
Nightshades (when cooked)	Sea vegetables
Red meat	Turmeric
Refined oils	
Refined sugars	

Anti-Aging

Here are some of the top signs of aging and their contributing factors:

1. Wrinkles: dehydration, inflammation, unhealthy fat deposits, poor circulation, and mineral deficiency

2. Atherosclerosis: inflammation

3. Aches and pains: inflammation, dehydration, mineral deficiency, and inorganic mineral deposits

4. Arthritis: inflammation, dehydration, inorganic mineral deposits, and acidic pH

5. Loss of bone density: acidic pH, mineral deficiency, and dehydration

6. Tooth decay: acidic pH and mineral deficiency

7. Loss of hearing: inorganic mineral deposits, inflammation, and poor circulation

8. Loss of vision: inorganic mineral deposits, inflammation, and poor circulation

9. Mental deterioration: inorganic mineral deposits, dehydration, inflammation, and poor circulation

10. Loss of sexual function: poor circulation, mineral deficiency, and dehydration

By embarking on a raw food detoxification program you will be well on your way to eliminating many of these factors and even slowing down some of the natural processes of aging.

FRESH FACT

Famous raw food enthusiasts include actor Woody Harrelson, comedian Robin Williams, and Apple CEO Steve Jobs.

The Least You Need to Know

- Raw food is uncooked, mostly plant-based whole food that contains numerous vital enzymes and nutrients.
- People who eat a raw food diet are often vegan and enjoy a healthy weight and good health in general.
- Detoxification is the removal or neutralization of toxic substances in the body and is a naturally occurring function.
- The body stores excess toxins in fat cells for your protection.
- The body may require help in eliminating a buildup of toxins that could otherwise result in a number of physical and psychological symptoms.

Our Toxic World

In This Chapter

- Getting to know your toxic enemies
- Noteworthy environmental toxins to avoid
- Understanding your detoxifying organs

In these pages, you'll learn about some of the basic toxins you may encounter—both environmentally and internally—that make a detox advisable. From pollution to pesticides to good old-fashioned stress, all types of toxins can become dangerous culprits of premature aging, weight gain, and degenerative disease. So it pays to know who and what you're up against.

Similarly, it's good to know who your friends are—and by that I mean those hardworking organs of the body that relentlessly strive to keep up with the plethora of toxins they face on a regular basis. These "organs of elimination" are the vital members of the anti-toxin team, and in this chapter you'll meet them briefly so you can become familiar with their roles in the process by better understanding what they do. I'm guessing you'll not only gain huge respect for them, but you may also commit to treating them better in the future by eliminating the entry of as many toxins as you can. In a world full of so much toxicity, every little bit helps.

Toxins 101

There's no escaping toxins. You can travel the globe and won't be able to find a single place on the surface of the planet that is free from this by-product of progress. There's no need to barricade yourself inside the house armed with a spray bottle full of bleach, however. Many toxins are simply part of our everyday life—a by-product of basic existence. Other toxins are manmade by-products of industry—some even global and far-reaching. Let's take a close look at these enemies who we hope to eliminate through our detoxification program.

FRESH FACT

Examples of "global toxins" include air pollution and water contamination in major cities, mercury found in fish, and jet fuel found in the breast milk of Eskimos.

Metabolic Waste

First is metabolic waste—a natural by-product of living. The body is constantly tearing itself down and rebuilding itself back up, and it's during this lifetime construction process that waste is created. The body is well prepared to deal with metabolic waste. Both *catabolic* and *anabolic processes* are normal body functions. When the body is given the proper fuel and building materials, this construction/deconstruction process usually occurs seamlessly. It's when the body becomes burdened by external toxins and is given inefficient fuel and inferior building materials that problems begin.

DEFINITION

Catabolic processes occur when old cells are broken down into smaller units and used for energy. **Anabolic processes** are when new cells are built using metabolized energy and raw materials.

Environmental Toxins

Our environment contains a host of toxins that are in the air, water, and objects around us. They can be as simple as mold or as complex as *polychlorinated biphenyls (PCBs)*. You can find them emanating from the building materials in your house or come across them in municipal water systems. Knowing the sources of the many environmental toxins in the area where you live enables you to take steps to minimize and eliminate them from your daily life. Often, it's possible to find safe alternatives for many of the environmental toxins we encounter, such as home cleaning products or gardening chemicals. Other times, they are not as easy to avoid—and citizens may need to advocate for their removal.

For example the use of bisphenol A (BPA), a compound used in plastics, has been banned for use in baby bottles in Canada and the European Union due to much concern after the release of a USDA study in 2010. Lobbying continues in the United States.

DEFINITION

Polychlorinated biphenyls (PCBs) are organic compounds once used in transformer and coolant fluids, but banned as a toxin by the U.S. Congress in 1979.

Top Environmental Toxins

Toxin	Potential Sources	Effects	Remedies and Safe Alternatives
Aluminum	Antiperspirants, metal cookware, antacids, aspirin, processed foods	Brain damage, skeletal defects	Avoid sources; use glass or cast-iron cookware
Arsenic	Water, pesticides, cigarettes, detergents	Cancer, heart disease, night blindness	Avoid sources; select sulfur-rich and fiber-rich foods; chelation therapy (heavy metal detox)
Asbestos	Ceiling insulation, drywall, floors, water pipes, heating ducts, toys, artificial fireplace logs	Cancer, scarring of lung tissue, mesothelioma (a form of cancer)	Avoid sources
Bisphenol A (BPA)	Water bottles, baby bottles, plastic wraps, food packaging	Abnormal fetal development	Avoid sources
Butylated hydroxyanisole (BHA)	Chewing gum, snack foods, diaper creams	Cancer	Avoid processed foods, read cream labels
Chlorine	Household cleaners, air near some industries (such as paper plants), drinking water (small amounts)	Sore throat, wheezing, fluid in lungs, rapid breathing, burns to skin/eyes, Reactive Airways Dysfunction Syndrome (RADS), which is a type of asthma	Water filtration; use chlorine-free household cleaners

continues

continued

Toxin	Potential Sources	Effects	Remedies and Safe Alternatives
Chloroform	Industrial effluent, municipal waste treatment plant discharges, hazardous waste sites and spills	Cancer, reproductive damage, birth defects, dizziness, fatigue, headache, liver and kidney damage	Avoid sources
Decabromo-diphenyl ether (DECA)—flame retardant	Electronics, furniture, carpets	Learning and memory deficits, hearing defects, possible fertility issues	Avoid sources
Dioxins	Animal fats: more than 95 percent of human exposure to these is from animal fats	Cancer, reproductive and developmental disorders, skin rashes, skin discoloration, chloracne (severe dermatitis with acne-like lesions), excessive body hair, mild liver damage	Reduce or eliminate animal product intake
Electromagnetic fields (EMFs)	Cell phones, electronic devices, microwaves, radio towers, high-tension power lines	Diabetes, cancer, endocrine imbalances	Limit exposure, unplug devices when not in use, rearrange living space to avoid direct contact, use EMF protection devices
Fluoride	Toothpaste, tap water, dental visits	Neurotoxins, cancer risk	Avoid sources; use distilled water and fluoride-free toothpaste
Lead	Plumbing, paint	Brain development, infertility, seizures, coma, death	Water filtration, distilled water, chelation therapy
Mercury	Dental fillings, fish	Brain damage, kidney damage, abnormal fetal development	Chelation therapy; select cilantro, sea vegetables, and chlorella, algae for comparable fish nutrition

Toxin	Potential Sources	Effects	Remedies and Safe Alternatives
Mold/fungus	Buildings; foods, including peanuts, wheat, corn, and alcohol	Cancer, asthma, multiple sclerosis (MS), heart disease, diabetes	Ozone remediation, dehumidifier, air filtration
Oxybenzone	Sunscreens, lip balm, moisturizers	Hormone disruptor, low birth weight	Avoid sources
Parabens	Moisturizers, hair care, shaving creams	Hormone disruptor, cancer	Use paraben-free products
Perchlorate	Drinking water, soil, some vegetables	Thyroid inhibitor	Water filtration, using distilled water
Perfluorooctanoic acid (PFOA)	Tap water, nonstick pots and pans	Hormone disruptor, reproductive damage, Alzheimer's Disease	Avoid sources
Pesticides/herbicides	Water, non-organic produce, processed foods, meat, bug sprays, lawn sprays	Cancer, Parkinson's Disease, nerve damage, miscarriage, birth defects	Avoid sources, grow your own produce, consume organic foods
Polychlorinated biphenyls (PCBs)	Farm-raised salmon	Cancer, impaired fetal brain development	Avoid sources
Pthalates	Cosmetics, toys, plastic wrap, bottles, food containers, shampoo, shower curtains, detergents	Endocrine system damage, abnormal fetal development, hormone disruptor, liver cancer	Avoid sources
Volatile organic compounds (VOCs)	Water, carpeting, cleaning fluids, paints and varnishes, deodorants, cosmetics, dry cleaning, air fresheners, moth repellents	Cancer, eye/respiratory problems, headache, impaired memory	Avoid sources, ozone remediation, get house plants

Sources: "10 Environmental Toxins to Avoid," by Marie Oser, found at tinyurl.com/3sp3z6f; "The Hazards Lurking at Home," by Alice Park, found at tinyurl.com/3qjcfj4.

Our Food and Water

Unfortunately, even raw foods can be contaminated with toxic chemicals unless they were grown using organic or chemical-free farming practices. This is why you need to know where your produce is from and how it was treated and grown before it arrived on your table. Chemical fertilizers, pesticides, and herbicides are often used in growing conventional fruits, vegetables, grains, nuts, and seeds. These chemically intensive farming practices can be toxic to the consumer in two ways. First, many of the conventionally grown crops have toxic residue on them, which the consumer ends up eating. Second, runoff water from conventional farmlands can contaminate local water supplies.

Just as our bodies tend to accumulate toxins within their fat cells, so do the bodies of animals. Factory-farmed livestock raised on an unnatural diet of pesticide- and herbicide-laden grains can potentially end up with concentrate toxins within their bodies. These toxins end up in our food supply and eventually make their way into the bodies of consumers. This is one of the main reasons some vegetarians choose to abstain from eating meat. If you choose to eat meat, a less toxic alternative is to choose free-range livestock and organic certified meat sources.

Food can also be toxic in ways that are less obvious. The more a food is processed, the more its food value is compromised. Think of a raw potato versus a potato chip. When does a food become so toxic that it's no longer a food? If a study was done to answer that question and steps were taken to remove toxic foods from "food stores," the shelves of most grocery stores would be practically bare. More than 90 percent of the food in the grocery store is processed and ultimately void of enzymes and most nutrition. In addition, many of these foods are made with an array of toxic additives and preservatives.

Another less-obvious way in which food can be toxic is in how it has been prepared or cooked. Some methods of cooking are better than others, but all cooking destroys enzymes and affects the nutritional profile of foods. Frying and high-heat grilling are the cooking methods that are most detrimental to health. Temperature and duration are two factors that play an important role in the production of some of these toxic by-products of cooking. By the way, raw food avoids playing the guessing game with these toxins by eliminating them at the source. No cooking, no problem.

All About GMOs

Since their introduction in 1996, genetically modified (GM) foods have become a topic of concern. GM foods are created from plant or animal sources that have been genetically manipulated and changed. GMO stands for "genetically modified organism"; often, GM or GE (genetically engineered) is used to describe foods containing these unnatural ingredients. The end result is a laboratory creation that has traits and characteristics that were deemed desirable. GM foods pose a less-obvious threat to health, although it is one that is proving to be serious.

Only one human study has been published, but there have been numerous studies done with laboratory animals. The results of those tests all show that GMOs have a negative impact on health. Another telling source of the shocking effects from consuming GMO crops comes from farmers who feed their livestock GMO feed. Some of the effects seen in laboratories and from farmers are premature death, organ damage, cancer, and birth defects. In humans, GMOs have been suspected in causing a host of health challenges, including allergies, behavioral disorders, genetic changes to internal flora, and even irritable bowel syndrome (IBS).

During the raw food detox program, you will be abstaining from packaged, processed, and chemically grown foods. The recipes and ingredients listed are of the non-GMO variety. Keep in mind, however, that even after you have finished doing your detox program, you still can benefit from avoiding GMO foods.

In a paper by Jeffrey M. Smith, "Doctors Warn: Avoid Genetically Modified Food," the American Academy of Environmental Medicine (AAEM) called on doctors to educate the public about the risks of genetically modified (GM) foods. They called for a moratorium on GM foods, long-term independent studies, and labeling. AAEM's position paper focused on some serious health risks associated with GM food, including infertility, immune problems, accelerated aging, insulin regulation, and changes in major organs and the gastrointestinal system. They conclude, "There is more than a casual association between GM foods and adverse health effects. There is causation," as defined by recognized scientific criteria. "The strength of association and consistency between GM foods and disease is confirmed in several animal studies."

Energetic Toxins

Electromagnetic fields (EMFs) are the charged fields created by electricity and electrically powered objects in our environment. Everyday items such as computer screens, cell phones, alarm clocks, and indoor and outdoor electrical lighting give off EMFs. Major sources such as substations, power lines, cell phone towers, and transformers are some industrial-strength EMF generators that we're exposed to every day. Be cautious of proximity and duration of exposure to EMFs. Long-term exposure to high levels of EMFs have been proven to cause an array of health problems, such as cancer, birth defects, miscarriages, sterility, and brain tumors. But even low-level exposure can be an everyday concern, because every electric convenience is a potential source of EMF pollution.

Magnetic field strength is measured in *Gauss* units, with low levels (which we normally experience in our daily lives) measured in milli Gauss units (mG). In Chapter 21 we'll be looking at how you can measure the EMF levels in your home and ultimately protect yourself from EMF radiation.

DEFINITION

Gauss (G) units measure the intensity of magnetic fields and are named after the nineteenth-century German scientist and mathematician Carl Friedrich Gauss.

Radiation

World events like the 2011 earthquake and nuclear reactor meltdown in Fukishima, Japan, have brought the risk of radiation contamination in air, water, and food to the attention of the world. Low-level radiation poisoning is a real concern with repercussions that can potentially show up years later in the form of cancer. Radiation damages living tissue by creating free radicals, which in turn destroy or alter DNA and RNA. A diet high in antioxidant-rich foods is one form of protection from radiation damage, but there are also foods and supplements that have been shown to aid in the detoxification of radiation from the body.

Sea vegetables and miso are foods that aid in radiation detox. Sea vegetables are able to provide an abundance of antioxidants and chelate heavy metals from the body. Another bonus that sea vegetables offer is that they are great source of iodine, which is critical for proper thyroid function. In instances where radioactive iodine is a risk it is necessary to provide the body with ample amounts of safe iodine to prevent the thyroid from taking in the radioactive iodine. A diet rich in sea vegetables can help achieve this.

Iodine Content in Sea Vegetables

Source of Iodine	Amount of Iodine
Kombu, 1-inch piece	1,454 mcg
Hiziki, 1 tablespoon	786 mcg
Arame, 1 tablespoon	732 mcg
Kelp (marine coast), 1 tablespoon	595 mcg
Alaria (marine coast), 1 tablespoon	218 mcg
Agar agar, 1 tablespoon	120 mcg
Wakame, 1 tablespoon	82 mcg
Dulse (marine coast), 1 tablespoon	68 mcg
Nori, 1 sheet	40 mcg
Lavar (marine coast), 1 tablespoon	19 mcg

Unpasteurized miso is also great protection against radiation damage, and its effects have been documented in numerous studies. Other foods that combat radiation damage include the superfoods blue-green algae, spirulina, and chlorella.

Stress

Many would argue that stress—the physiological burden most humans experience on a daily basis—is the number one cause of aging and degenerative disease in the world. If you can master stress, you can master anything. Diet, exercise, and mental and spiritual practices are some of the ways we can do this—but more on that later in the book.

In terms of toxicity, stress causes oxidation in the body, taxes the body's reserve of antioxidants and nutrients, and changes the body's pH to a more acidic state. There is both a psychological and biological component to stress, and hormones play a large part. Stress begins in the mind, when an individual or animal responds to a perceived threat. Once the mind believes it is threatened, the biological components of stress kick in. This is the "fight or flight" component of stress in which the heart rate increases, adrenaline is released, and senses are heightened.

Other responses to stress are negativity, moodiness, irritability, procrastination, depression, anti-social behavior, overeating and not eating, sleeping too much, and sleeping too little as well, as many other reactions. Interestingly, certain foods can contribute to stress as well, while others can help alleviate it. We'll learn more about stress and the role that raw food detox can play in alleviating it in Chapter 4, but for now, know that there's an internal toxin you may actually have the ability to dramatically control.

Organs of Elimination

Now that we know a bit about the types of toxins we are up against—as well as the basic two-phase process of eliminating them (that we saw in Chapter 1)—let's take a closer look at the organs of the body that are directly involved in this very serious detox activity. Each of them plays a vital role in filtering, expelling, deconstructing, and eliminating toxins from the body. When a single member of this eliminative team is compromised, the entire team suffers—and so does the body. A good-quality detox plan provides the needed support to enable these organs to get the job done and keep the toxins flowing out so that health can flow in.

The Bowels

Many people don't pay much attention to their bowels. Digestive topics are not always popular, and many of us often dismiss annoying symptoms of irregularity or indigestion as unimportant. Ignoring the state of your bowels, however, can prove a costly mistake for health. It has even been suggested that the condition of the bowels may be key in understanding one's state of health or underlying disease. It has also been suggested that the cleanliness of any tissue in the body depends on the condition of the bowels, which is a very important point in the context of detoxification. Here's why.

Going back to the house analogy in referring to the body, the bowels represent the foundation of the house. This foundation, like the bowels, is often overlooked because it's tucked away and out of sight. A diet and lifestyle that neglects the needs of the bowels can result in the weakening of the foundation upon which the body is built. Once the foundation of a house is compromised, it is only a matter of time before the integrity of the rest of the structure is compromised. That's why nutrient-dense, fiber-rich, alkalizing, and hydrating whole foods are so critical for health and wellness—but more on that in our next chapter.

Further, years of toxicity and abuse tend to accumulate in the bowels. It would be nice if eating a papaya could make it all go away, but it won't. The need for fasting, colon hydrotherapy, and enemas is often required to get the bowels back on track and functioning at their peak. Once the bowels are functioning properly, a good diet and nutrition along with a healthy lifestyle will take care of things quite well.

The Skin

Did you know that the skin is your largest organ of elimination? Every inch of your body is covered with pores, and these tiny openings allow waste to be excreted from the body. When the skin is glowing, your health is showing—but when the "glow don't show," there's trouble below! Skin conditions such as acne, rashes, and eczema are a signal that there may be a toxic burden on the body. There are different methods to optimize the skin's detoxifying abilities. The skin loves sun and fresh air. Skin brushing, exfoliating, steam baths, and exercise (as well as, of course, an excellent diet) help stimulate the eliminative power of the skin.

The Lungs

The lungs inhale about 11,000 liters of air and exhale a combination of oxygen, carbon dioxide, and metabolic toxins every day. The lungs, like the heart, are an organ partially composed of muscle. Among their functions, the lungs are responsible for cleansing the air by removing particles via cilia located on the walls of all the passageways. When they're overloaded, excess mucous, coughing, and a number of respiratory diseases can begin to develop. The practice of deep breathing as well as other yogic breathing exercises can strengthen the lungs and increase their detoxification potential—and a number of raw foods have been shown to be instrumental in maintaining healthy lung function.

The Kidneys

While the lungs process the air we take in, the kidneys process liquids. One of the main functions of the kidneys is also to purify our blood. The kidneys rarely get a break, because they are filtering the foods and liquids we take in on a constant basis. Anything we can do to help our friendly kidneys is important in maintaining health. They particularly love pure water, but there are also hydrating foods and herbal teas that support kidney function (which we'll be making in Chapter 15).

The Liver

Some give the liver the crown for detoxing the body while others bestow that honor upon the bowels. There's no arguing that both are critical for detoxifying the body. The liver does get the prize for being the largest internal organ and the largest gland. The liver contributes to detoxification by neutralizing toxins or storing them. Aside from storage and detoxification, the liver decomposes red blood cells, emulsifies fats for digestion, makes plasma protein, stores glycogen, and produces hormones. It is clearly the hardest-working organ in the body.

One of the particularly amazing things about the liver is its regenerative properties. Twenty-five percent of a functioning liver can regenerate itself into a new, fully functioning liver (with proper care and nutrition, of course). Although the liver is susceptible to a number of ailments, including hepatitis, fatty liver, and cirrhosis, it is very resilient and benefits exceedingly well from a healthy diet.

The Lymphatic System

The blood that travels through our arteries and veins usually gets top billing when it comes to vital liquids circulating throughout the body, while the lymphatic system is often overlooked. But lymphatic liquid—a clear fluid whose main purpose is transporting *lymphocytes* throughout the body—is particularly important when it comes to the topic of toxins. These guys deal with invasive cells and organisms such as tumors as well as bacteria and viruses. Lymphatic liquid also works as an intermediary with the blood circulatory system by transporting nutrients in and waste out.

> **DEFINITION**
>
> **Lymphocytes** are the special forces of the immune system, consisting of natural killer cells (NK cells), T cells, and B cells.

The organs that make up the lymphatic system are the tonsils, thymus gland, spleen, and bone marrow. Other components of this feeding, cleaning, and defensive system are lymph nodes and lymph vessels. Lymphatic liquid flows from the extremities toward the heart in this one-way system. The lymphatic system doesn't have a pump like the heart to keep its fluids moving, however. It relies on the contractions of the lymph organs and muscle contractions. Movement, especially exercise, helps circulate the lymphatic fluid and is very supportive of its proper functioning. Keeping this system working well and removing the stress of excess toxins will go a long way toward keeping the entire group of elimination organs working efficiently and smoothly.

The Least You Need to Know

- Toxins can be external, such as pollution, or generated internally through metabolic functions.
- There are a growing number of environmental toxins that we need to watch out for and try to avoid.
- The main parts of the body involved in detoxification are the bowels, skin, lungs, kidneys, liver, and lymphatic system.
- Successful detoxification requires all parts of the body to function at peak level.
- By providing quality fuel and nutrition such as that found in a raw food diet, you can help your body naturally detoxify.

Why Raw Food Detox Works

In This Chapter

- Achieving proper balance
- Amazing enzymes
- The importance of food combining

In this chapter, you'll discover the reasons why raw food works for detoxifying the body, rejuvenating your insides, revitalizing your outsides, and helping you reach your ideal weight.

From understanding the importance of balancing the acidity and alkalinity in your system to putting to use some amazing enzymes available to you in raw food, you'll get why its vital to detox yourself using the advice in this book.

Keeping you glowing and beautiful on the outside is only the beginning. Your insides will be smiling as well.

Balance Restoration

Health is a balancing act in many ways. Many internal and external factors come into play—toxins to eliminate, nutrition to assimilate, water to hydrate, air to oxygenate, fiber to evacuate, and exercise to invigorate—and raw food detox can take care of a good portion of these issues. It's amazing what the body can do once it's given the foods it craves for great health.

Acid and Alkaline

You may remember acids, bases, and the pH scale as a topic of discussion in chemistry class. The pH of an acid or base substance refers to the scale used to measure acidity and alkalinity (basicity). Just about all substances have a rating, and not surprisingly, the human body and its fluids also have distinct pH ratings, which can be important indicators of one's health and wellness.

Specifically, the scale measures the concentration of dissolved hydronium ions (H_3O^+) in a solution. The range of the scale is from 1 (extremely acidic) to 14 (extremely alkaline), with 7 being neutral. The pH of one's blood can be a tell-tale sign of imbalances in the body. The ideal pH for human blood is slightly alkaline, between 7.35–7.45. When the blood pH is higher or lower than that range, a person's health is usually compromised—and he or she may develop conditions referred to as *acidosis* or *alkalosis*.

DEFINITION

An overly acidic condition in the human body is referred to as *acidosis,* while an overly alkaline condition is referred to as *alkalosis.*

The exact pH ratings of body fluids tend to hover around the 7 (or neutral) mark. Normal ratings for common body fluids are as follows:

>   Blood = 7.4
>
>   Gastric juice = 0.7
>
>   Urine = 6.0–6.4
>
>   Pancreatic juice = 8.1
>
>   Cerebrospinal fluid = 7.3
>
>   Saliva = 6.4–7.0
>
>   Semen = 7.5

Usually, the blood pH imbalance will produce symptoms. Typically, a condition of acidosis (a blood pH of less than 7.35) can result in headaches, sleepiness, confusion, loss of consciousness, coma, shortness of breath, coughing, arrhythmia, increased heart rate, nausea, vomiting, seizures, weakness, or diarrhea. Common symptoms of alkalosis (a blood pH greater than 7.45), on the other hand, are irritability, muscle twitches, muscle spasms, and muscular weakness. For the most part, the condition of acidosis is much more common than alkalosis, as the body naturally tends toward a more acid state.

To maintain proper pH of bodily fluids—especially the blood—the body will beg, borrow, and steal minerals to achieve this balance. This is called buffering, and it is done using electrolytes, which are electrically charged solutions. Calcium, magnesium, and potassium are the body's major electrolyte minerals.

The balancing act the body plays with pH through buffering can throw off the other systems of the body. For example, acidic conditions are normally remedied by drawing upon the body's reserve of the alkalizing minerals. The major alkalizing minerals are calcium, iron, potassium, magnesium, manganese, and sodium. The bones act to buffer the blood's pH by offering its stores of alkaline salts in the case of acidity. When this occurs, stores of calcium are pulled from the bones—and, in many cases, from the teeth. An acidic diet (composed mostly of meat, dairy, and processed foods) constantly draws upon these reserves, leading to health challenges such as osteoporosis or tooth loss.

This is just one example of how a pH imbalance can affect the body. But by eating raw foods, which are primarily alkaline, you can avoid many of these possibilities. Because the raw food detox program consists of predominantly alkalizing foods, your body will be provided with concentrated nutrients in a form that's easy for it to use. In fact, if you are eating raw foods on a regular basis, it is likely that the need to balance the body's pH will become less of an issue.

FRESH FACT

The acid and alkaline way of eating is nothing new. Hippocrates was prescribing a healing diet of 80 percent alkaline foods more than 2,000 years ago, and his patients didn't have to cope with our abundant levels of environmental toxins, processed foods, and chemical additives!

A Partial List of Alkaline and Acid-Forming Foods

Alkaline-Forming	Neutral	Acid-Forming
All fruits except blueberries, cranberries, and plums	Fresh butter, unsalted	Alcohol
All greens (kale, spinach, lettuce)	Margarine	Artificial sweeteners
All sprouts	Oils	Blueberries
Amaranth	Raw cow's milk	Brazil nuts
Apple cider vinegar	Raw cream	Cranberries
Fresh herbs	Whey	Dried coconut
Millet	Yogurt	Macadamia nuts
Miso		Meat
Nutritional yeast		Most cooked foods
Olive oil		Olives, pickled
Quinoa		Pasteurized dairy products
Raw goat's milk		Pecans
Sea salt		Plums
Sea vegetables		Processed foods
Sesame seeds		Prunes
Soy products		Pumpkin seeds
Sprouted grains		Rice
Sweet brown-rice vinegar		Sunflower seeds
Wheatgrass		Unsprouted grains
		Walnuts

Bacteria and Flora

We're outnumbered. Would you believe that more bacteria are populating our bodies than our own cells? More than one trillion live in and on us. These living organisms are involved in a life-supporting, symbiotic relationship with our bodies. Ideal health can be achieved when the perfect ratio of nearly 500 different strains of bacteria are cultivated and nurtured in the body. These microbes are sensitive to light, heat, moisture, pH, toxins, and the food we consume. They are part of the ongoing balancing act known as personal health and wellness.

When an imbalance of good and bad bacteria occurs, so does the increased possibility of illness. If imbalances continue, a disease state can set in. The many strains of healthy internal bacteria are called probiotics, and the majority of them live in our large intestines. The balancing game in our gut, once again, comes down to pH. When the proper pH is established in the bowels, our internal flora (healthy bacteria) aid in digestion, produce B vitamins and amino acids, and prevent the growth of pathogenic bacteria. A pH near and higher than 7.0 is best. This neutral to slightly alkaline environment is where the digestive enzymes of the bowel can function best. Raw foods are key to keeping the balance—not only for the fluids and organs of the body but also for our internal flora. Greens and foods containing chlorophyll, such as plants, are ideal for feeding our healthy bacteria—and a raw food diet is naturally rich in green chlorophyll-containing foods.

FRESH FACT

Fermented foods are an ally in establishing and maintaining a well-balanced internal environment of healthy bacteria and flora. These foods are unpasteurized, fermented vegetables, such as sauerkraut and kimchi; fermented bean paste, such as miso; raw apple cider vinegar; and fermented beverages, such as kombucha.

Antibiotics are effective in doing one thing: killing bacteria. Antibiotics don't discriminate; rather, they kill the good bacteria with the bad, leaving no one spared. In cases of infection, antibiotics may be necessary to prevent severe infection and death. The periodic use and abuse of antibiotics, however, can contribute to long-term health issues and the development of antibiotic-resistant bacteria (superbugs). After taking antibiotics, it is critical to reestablish healthy bacteria in the intestines. If this isn't actively pursued, bacteria will reestablish itself on a first-come, first-served basis. Which bacteria (healthy or unhealthy) gains dominance is established by body pH and the bacteria that are reintroduced first. Raw food detoxification can help restore this balance and help deter the growth of unhealthy bacteria.

Hydration

Water is one of the most overlooked and underappreciated health foods. Technically, it has no calories or nutrient content. Like oxygen, though, which is calorie free, we can't live without it. While in the womb, our bodies go from being made up of 97 percent water to 80 percent at birth. As we age, the percentage of water we contain decreases. An adult's body consists of around 67 percent water. A 2 percent decrease in water in the body can impair thinking and energy levels. Larger drops in water content can result in serious health problems, while drops greater than 10 percent can result in death.

Dehydration statistics suggest that up to 75 percent of individuals in developed nations are chronically dehydrated. Chronic dehydration can contribute to arthritis, allergies, constipation, depression, insomnia, fatigue, headaches, high blood pressure, high cholesterol, weight gain, overeating, accelerated aging, and back pain. Wow—can you imagine that just by drinking the recommended eight eight-ounce glasses of water a day, you could alleviate or reverse these conditions? It makes sense, because the inner environment of our bodies is bathed in water. All the vital systems of the body use this liquid life to transport both nutrients and waste material. If you're dehydrated, it's like trying to sail a boat during low tide. You end up stuck in the mud.

As mentioned in Chapter 2, quality of water is just as important as quantity. A portion of the 64-ounce daily water requirement can be offset by eating water-dense foods. Raw fruits and vegetables are ideal for hydration. The water quality in chemical-free produce grown in nutrient-rich soil is just what the body wants and needs. Consuming 60 percent–100 percent of your calories from raw foods and drinking plenty of pure water is another part of the equation for creating optimal health.

Hydrochloric Acid (HCl)

Hydrochloric acid (HCl) is a key player in proper digestion and optimal health. HCl is a strong acid with a pH of 0.5 that is critical for protein digestion, which takes place in the lower stomach. HCl also activates pepsin, the protein-splitting enzyme, by dropping the pH in the lower stomach.

When the body is deficient in alkaline minerals, specifically sodium (Na), the body refuses to produce HCl. This is for self-preservation, because sodium is necessary for protecting/buffering the stomach from the extremely acidic HCl. Weak HCl secretion results in a higher pH in the stomach, which results in undigested proteins—and, worst of all, the survival of potentially harmful organisms (parasites) and bacteria, such as salmonella and E. coli, which would not survive in the normally highly acidic conditions in the lower stomach. So you can see why a deficiency in one nutrient has a cascading effect that influences all the body's systems. A raw food detox, high in alkalizing raw foods, can help alleviate this deficiency.

Plant-Based Nutrition

Raw foods come to the rescue in the case of vitamin and mineral deficiencies and imbalances of internal flora. Raw and living foods typically contain higher concentrations of a full spectrum of bioavailable nutrients, which are those vitamins and minerals that can be absorbed and used by the body. A cooked or processed food may contain x amount of a nutrient, such as calcium listed on the ingredient list of a processed cereal. This might look good on paper, but the body doesn't read labels—it reads molecular structure. If those nutrients are synthetic and/or inorganic, they are practically useless. Although plants can consume inorganic nutrients, such as the minerals in rock dust, we are unable to utilize them in this form. But plants are thankfully able to turn these inorganic minerals into organic compounds, which we can consume and utilize. All mammals get their organic minerals and compounds from plants, either directly or indirectly (even if they are carnivores), by eating animals that have eaten plant substances.

Vitamins and Minerals

Organic minerals and compounds manage the pH of the body. These minerals are organic because they're bound to a carbon atom and derived from plant or animal sources. An example of an organic versus inorganic compound is sea salt ($NaCl$) versus laboratory-made salt ($NaCl$). Both have the same chemical equation, but they are far from being the same. Sea salts aren't made up only of sodium (Na) and chlorine (Cl). An array of trace minerals in sea salt makes it different, and the beneficial properties of organic minerals and compounds can be altered by heat. When sea salt is sun-dried, it retains its beneficial properties—but when it is kiln-dried at a high temperature, it becomes inorganic and unusable by the body. The same can be said of nutritionally fortified processed foods. Just because the box lists calcium, sodium, and various vitamins doesn't mean the body can actually use them.

Raw foods contain a full spectrum of vitamins and minerals in proper ratios. Nature has gone to the trouble of balancing the nutrients in raw foods in a way that chemists and scientists have yet to figure out how to replicate. For example, studies have shown that the calcium in supplements taken alone is not easily assimilated into the body, especially if it's inorganic. It has also been shown that other trace minerals play a critical role in proper absorption of calcium in the body: magnesium, manganese, boron, zinc, and copper. Are there other factors to consider? Most likely. What are the proper ratios? Who knows. Raw foods remove all the guesswork and scientific speculation.

When you get vitamins and minerals from raw foods, you are guaranteed to receive them in a form that's ideal for your body. For special cases, you can consume specific foods that have a high concentration of nutrients that your body may need. For example, kale—which is a fibrous leafy green that is often boiled—is an amazing nutrient-dense food even after its nutritional profile has been compromised by cooking. Raw kale can be prepared or juiced, and all of its concentrated nutrition is maintained. Kale is alkalizing and anti-inflammatory and contains all the essential amino acids required to make it a complete protein. It also has a full spectrum of vitamins and minerals—some way beyond recommended allowances. And the fiber in kale is ideal for cleansing and proper elimination, which brings us to our next raw food advantage: fiber.

Fabulous Fiber

Roughage moves the world, and plant fiber is the best that nature has to offer. The fiber from unadulterated raw vegetables is tops. Fruits contain a great deal of soluble fiber—an essential nutrient. Soluble fibers absorb water and create a moist gel that helps keep things moving in your body.

Fruit skins consist of insoluble fiber, while the flesh contains soluble fiber such as pectin. Soluble fiber serves several purposes. It has a binding effect that helps lower cholesterol; it's involved with sugar absorption, helping normalize blood sugar; and it acts as a prebiotic, which feeds healthy bacteria in the large intestine. Vegetables and leafy greens contain a large amount of insoluble fiber, which acts as a bulking agent and helps move foods rapidly through the digestive tract.

Bran, the fibrous outer layer of grain, has been hailed as a great source of insoluble fiber by purveyors of processed foods. Although bran is indeed a source of insoluble fiber that can provide for regularity of the bowels, it's arguable that it is as good a source as it's often touted. Bran is by-product of processing whole grains into less-nutritious and more stable products, such as white flour and white rice. It was originally discarded or fed to livestock. Bran is not an ideal fiber for human consumption because of its rigid and sharp structure. Bran, along with whole grains, has a tendency to irritate the delicate lining of the stomach and the bowels. This is one reason why grains may cause allergic reactions in many individuals. Long-term irritation of the bowels can cause conditions known as Inflammatory Bowel Disease (IBD) and Irritable Bowel Syndrome (IBS), which are indications that the body is responding to inflammatory foods. The fiber in raw fruits and vegetables doesn't do this. Raw, plant-based sources, aside from grains, provide a variety of soluble and insoluble fiber to meet the needs of the body.

The Magic of Enzymes

We are aware of the necessity of vitamins and minerals for health, but without enzymes you might as well try to run your car without fuel. Sometimes referred to as the "blue-collar workers" of the living world, enzymes are at the core of all living processes. If life and death are a grand puppet show, enzymes are pulling the strings.

With age, as well as constant use and periodic abuse, the body's enzyme activity decreases and eventually ceases. Numerous lab studies have shown a direct correlation between enzymatic action and overall health. This is especially apparent when comparing enzyme concentration and the vitality of an adult to that of a child. The enzymes from the adult are less concentrated and less active than those of a child. Why? The detrimental effects of eating cooked foods factor into results found in a laboratory. When an animal eats its natural diet of enzyme-rich raw foods, enzyme activity and concentration is nearly identical between young and old.

Enzymes as Life Force

Enzymes are composed of proteins and organic compounds, but that's not all. The key to enzymes is the life force that powers them. Because they are indeed "alive," these workers are able to act as catalysts and initiators for all vital processes occurring in living organisms.

Like any worker in a complex system, enzymes are directed by the needs of a higher organism. Enzymes within a plant seed have the purpose of supporting the growth and propagation of that seed. Enzymes within a person's digestive system disassemble food into easily assimilated components. Enzymes can remain intact and be utilized even if the host organism is no longer alive. Animals and humans alike take advantage of this fact when consuming enzyme-rich foods.

There are three types of enzymes: metabolic, digestive, and food. The human body has a supply of both digestive and metabolic enzymes, while food enzymes are taken into the body when consuming raw and living foods. Enzymes are a precious currency in a healthy, living body, and thousands of different types of enzymes have been identified. Deficiencies of enzymes can be a precursor to a serious collapse of the body's health.

Metabolic enzymes initiate and maintain all metabolic activities in the body. It takes hundreds of enzymes to carry out the body's metabolic processes, which are activities such as expiration of carbon dioxide from inhaled oxygen or the processing of glucose into energy.

Digestive enzymes take care of food digestion. The three main digestive enzymes break down the three macro nutrients (carbohydrates, proteins, and fats) into smaller, usable forms:

- Amylase takes care of digesting carbohydrates.
- Protease handles proteins.
- Lipase dismantles fats.

Each of the digestive enzymes has an ideal pH in which it functions. At one time, it was thought that foods were chewed up and swallowed and an even mixture of all the digestive enzymes was excreted to create a big enzyme—"food soup" within the stomach. This is not the case. Foods are digested systematically, and certain food combinations are more ideal for optimal digestion than others. This is the basis for food combining. There is a simple science to eating that once was instinctive, and following simple food-combining principles (discussed later in this chapter) can result in some amazing results.

Raw Chemical Reactions

Food enzymes exist outside the body and are part of the magic of living, raw foods. Some food enzymes regulate the ripening process while others break down the foods or organisms once they are past their prime. Within nuts, seeds, grains, and legumes, there are enzymes involved in the dramatic growth processes that take place to generate a new plant.

Enzyme inhibitors prevent seeds from sprouting while inside the fruit or under less-than-ideal conditions. These chemicals are deactivated with temperature and moisture changes. Some of these enzyme inhibitors can be dangerous if consumed in excess, such as trypsin inhibitors, which are in high concentration in soybeans, causing gastric upset and even near toxic reactions. Soaking, sprouting, and cooking deactivate enzyme inhibitors, but only soaking and sprouting leave the beneficial enzymes intact.

The human body has a single stomach with two sections: upper and lower. The upper section secretes no enzymes or acid and has no *peristalsis* activity. This inactive, enzyme-less upper stomach provides a place for the enzymes within foods (raw foods) to begin digestion of carbohydrates, proteins, and fats.

DEFINITION

Peristalsis is the wavelike contractions that move food along the digestive tract.

The digestion of starches actually begins in the mouth with the alkaline enzyme secretion ptyalin (amylase). This digestion continues in the food enzyme (upper) stomach for about one hour. Upon leaving the upper stomach, the protein-splitting enzyme pepsin is secreted—but due to the alkaline pH of the upper stomach, it isn't activated until it settles into the lower stomach, where hydrochloric acid has dropped the lower stomach's pH so that protein digestion can continue. Enzyme-less cooked and processed food sits for at least an hour, putrefying and fermenting in the upper stomach. Toxins are created as a by-product—one of the reasons for gas and bloating.

By taking advantage of the external food enzymes present in raw foods, you can optimize your digestion and spare the body its limited reserve of much-needed enzymes. The body can tell when you're eating cooked foods versus raw foods and manages its enzyme reserves accordingly. Eating raw foods means that the body needs to produce only a minimal amount of digestive enzymes. This is a huge relief for the body systems involved in enzyme production. When fewer enzymes are used for digesting food, then more enzymes can be used for other maintenance and upkeep of the body. By optimizing the allocation of the body's resources, chronic conditions can be dealt with and the systems of the body can be strengthened. Raw foods are a win-win combination.

Heat in excess of 118° Fahrenheit destroys enzymes. So, cooking destroys enzymes, heat processing destroys enzymes, and even freezing destroys enzymes. Enzymes should be treated like gold—like the currency of life. Invest in enzymes, and your returns will be health and longevity.

Food Combining

Food combining takes into account the body's physiological response to specific types of foods. Dr. Herbert M. Shelton is regarded as the father of food combining. He noticed that certain foods require less time to transit the stomach than others, and also that foods such as starches require alkaline digestive juices while proteins require digestive juices that are acidic.

Appendix B provides a comprehensive chart for food combining, so be sure to refer to it often. If a person respects the laws of food combining, the body responds in kind with easy and efficient digestion, assimilation, and elimination. If, on the other hand, dietary violations of combining occur, the body responds with digestive distress, poor assimilation, and eliminative challenges.

Food combining for raw and cooked foods is similar in concept, yet they differ slightly due to the less prevalent amount of complex carbohydrates (starch) that are part of a raw food diet. For simplicity's sake we'll explore raw food combining principles in greater detail than cooked food combining principles. I encourage you to investigate this topic in further detail on your own, however.

The One-Lane Digestive Expressway

Consider your digestive system as an expressway for the foods you eat. Each type of food—fruits, vegetables, nuts, seeds, dairy, meat, processed foods, etc—represents a type of vehicle. Some are sports cars while others are trucks, and some shouldn't even be allowed in the road. The digestive expressway is a single "no passing lane"—this is rule number one of food combining. With this in mind, ideally the fastest-moving foods would always enter the expressway first to prevent slowdowns and traffic jams.

Water passes through the digestive system in a matter of minutes, and foods high in water content do the same. The simpler the food, the faster it digests; the more complex the food, the longer it takes to digest. Fruits, especially melons, are the fastest-digesting foods. Watermelon can move from the stomach to the small intestines in under 30 minutes. Other water-rich fruits take closer to an hour. The lower water content a raw food has, the longer it takes to digest, so dehydrated fruits require more time in the stomach than fresh fruits.

Once you introduce cooked or dense foods, digestion time dramatically increases. When a fast-digesting food like fresh fruit gets caught behind a slow-digesting food like cooked animal protein you get a digestive traffic jam, the results of which are indigestion, gas, and bloating. This is a result of the fruit sugars fermenting while they're waiting for the more complex proteins to be digested. Problems like these can be avoided by eating "fast and simple foods" first and then following them with more complex foods.

Proper Eating Order

Give the sports car room to move: 20 to 30 minutes is enough of a head start. Do not consume juices or water with meals because it will dilute your digestive fire. If your meal is too difficult to consume without water or liquids, you probably shouldn't be eating it.

After water and juices are consumed first, the following list provides a good rule of thumb for eating foods in their proper order:

- **Melons.** These are the fastest digesting of all the fruits. Eat melons on their own and allow 30 minutes before eating any other foods.

- **Fruits.** There are four categories of fruits: starchy, sub-acid, acid, and sweet (see Appendix B for more about this). All fruits combine well with other fruits that are within their same groups, as well as adjacent groups. For example, sub-acid is fine with acid, but not fine with sweet. Don't leap frog groups, though, or you'll end up with indigestion. Ripe is the key consideration here. If a fruit isn't fully ripened, then it may be more starch or acid than simple sugar. An unripe banana is starchy rather than sweet and it makes you constipated, while a ripe banana is sweet and supports elimination.

- **Leafy greens, vegetable sprouts, and celery.** These guys combine well with most everything, but don't pair them with fast-digesting fruits. Apples, pears, and berries can be added to salads in small amounts without any problem. Greens are an ideal partner with proteins and fats. That's why salad dressings work so well on salads.

- **Starchy vegetables.** Keep these guys away from proteins at all costs. Avoid combining them with fruits, especially acid fruits. Starchy vegetables do well with leafy greens, sprouts, and avocado.

- **Sprouted grains and beans.** These guys are predominantly starches. They combine well with leafy greens. Sprouted beans and grains consist of both starch and protein, however, which may explain why some people find them on occasion to be hard to digest.

- **Protein.** Keep the proteins in nuts, seeds, and olives away from starches. This isn't very difficult to do when eating raw foods. (It is far more difficult to control when consuming cooked meals.) Combine raw proteins with leafy greens, fats, non-starchy vegetables, non-sweet fruits, lemon, lime and vegetable sprouts.

- **Fats.** Fats do best and combine well with everything that proteins combine with.

In addition to the points in the preceding list, remember that neither fats nor proteins combine well with sweet fruits. This is a heartbreaker when it comes to raw desserts. Using dry fruits to make desserts seems to take the edge off of this food-combining faux pas. One thing to keep in mind, though, is an improperly food-combined raw dessert is most likely better for you than a dessert that is made with processed and cooked ingredients.

Avoid the Protein and Starch Pileup

The second rule for food combining is violated on a daily basis in the cooked food world. The standard fare that represents the pinnacle of nostalgic American eating is in violation of this law: Do not consume starches and proteins at the same meal. See what I mean? This flies in the face of the "meat and potatoes" battle cry that's at the heart of a variety of cultural cuisines.

Here are some examples of standard protein/starch combos in our culture:

- Steak/baked potato
- Burger/fries and bun
- Fish/chips
- Hot dog/bun

- Sandwich meat/bread
- Chicken/rice
- Fish/rice
- Meat toppings/pizza crust
- Meatballs/pasta

Protein-rich foods are easy to identify because they're typically flesh foods. The starches that accompany them are less obvious but easily identified once you know what to look for. Starches are complex carbohydrates, which is just a way of saying "not simple sugars." Grains, corn, root vegetables, cooked beans, and rice make up the basic list of starches. Many of these foods are inedible raw and require cooking to make them palatable.

Breads, cooked potatoes, and rice are the most common starches consumed and they're often partnered with animal protein. The problem with this combination is that proteins require an acid pH for digestion while starches require an alkaline pH. Upon consuming protein and starch in the same meal we have an immediate conflict of pH. The result of this conflict is that alkaline and acid digestive juices end up neutralizing each other, which results in only partial digestion of both foods. Meats putrefy and starches ferment in the digestive tract, forcing the body to expend large amounts of energy and resources to eliminate the toxins created. The science behind this is very simple and the widespread violation of this food combining rule and its repercussions are easily observed.

The number one over-the-counter drug sold in the United States is digestive aids. Just turn the television on during dinnertime and make note of the commercials for antacids, gas relief, and constipation. Makes you wonder what factor contributes to this nationwide need for digestive aids? The protein/starch digestive disaster is the first place to start looking.

This combining problem is easily remedied by substituting vegetables for either the protein or starch in the meal. Instead of chicken and rice, have a chicken salad. Instead of meat and potatoes, have steamed broccoli and potatoes. With raw foods, animal protein and starches aren't part of the dietary equation so this rule doesn't cause much of a problem.

A protein rule that applies to both raw and cooked camps is to only eat a single protein food at any one time. A variety meat buffet is an express ticket to indigestion and other potential long-term complications. With raw foods, keep recipes simple by only using a single type of nut, seed, or protein powder, such as spirulina. Simplicity can literally save your stomach and possibly your life.

Tools for Aiding Digestion

If you haven't noticed yet, enzymes are key to raw food detox and they are key to healthy living. This message is worth repeating: *Enzymes = Life.* If your food is lifeless there is a remedy; take digestive enzyme capsules with your meals. Digestive enzyme supplements are beneficial when eating either cooked meals or raw meals. I eat close to 100 percent raw and I still make a point to eat enzyme capsules with most of my meals. Enzymes are simple and effective in aiding the digestion process, and most people can use all the help they can get.

Some enzyme shopping tips:

- Look for digestive enzymes at health-food stores and also online. Compare price, quantity, concentration, and variety of enzymes in the different brands.
- Enzymes are measured by potency, not weight. You will notice letters like "HUT," "DU," and "ALU" after each enzyme listed. This is the potency per unit. The higher the number the more potent that enzyme is.
- Use the potency as a benchmark when comparing enzymes.
- Purchase only organic-certified and vegan enzymes.

Some quality enzyme brands to check out are LifeGive HHI-Zyme, Enzymedica DigestGold, and Dr. Howell's Digestive Enzymes.

Keep enzymes handy especially when dining out, visiting friends, or traveling. Enzymes are relatively heat stable when dried, so you can leave them in your car or carry them in your backpack or purse without any concerns.

Another simple way to optimize digestion at meal times is to consume fermented foods with your meals. Unpasteurized sauerkraut, kimchi, and miso can add a boost to your digestive capabilities. Fermented foods are acidic, so they do not combine well with starches. I like to add them to green salads or use them to kick up the flavor factor in nori rolls or collard wraps.

Remember that although they aid digestion, enzyme supplements and fermented foods do not allow you to violate food-combining rules. Listen to your body and respect its responses to your food-combining choices.

The Least You Need to Know

- Raw food helps balance the pH of the body's fluids, preventing acidosis, which can be the cause of many conditions and illnesses.
- Raw food keeps healthy bacteria present in the digestive tract in good amounts, while maintaining the body's hydration, and keeping hydrochloric acid at proper levels.
- The nutrition obtained from plant-based, raw foods is plentiful in vitamins, minerals, and both soluble and insoluble fiber.
- Enzymes are extremely important substances for optimal nutrition and can be destroyed in cooking, heating, and freezing.
- Following the rules of food combining will guarantee healthy digestion and good overall well-being.

Calling in Reinforcements

In This Chapter

- Exercise as an adjunct detoxer
- Help with toxic elimination through the skin
- All about colon hydrotherapy

The food that goes into your mouth and its assimilation is only part of the detox and health equation. Yes, changing your diet is a powerful way to transform your health—but when it is combined with a variety of other health-supporting activities, the road to radiance becomes a blur as you rapidly move toward your health goals. Exercise supports health, but there are also other simple activities, such as skin brushing, that take only minutes yet have long-lasting effects on wellness.

In this chapter, we take a close look at some activities and habits that you can adopt to reinforce your program and help you achieve optimum results.

Exercise

What simple act can counter depression, kick-start your metabolism, offset blood sugar imbalances, and aid in detoxification? If you guessed exercise, give yourself a raw treat. The benefits of exercise are undeniable. Back in the hunter-and-gatherer days, no one jogged unless they were chasing something or being chased—and a stair machine was just a long walk up a mountainside. Clearly, forms of exercise and the equipment we use have evolved along with technology, but the basic concept has always remained the same—exercising the body is good for health and well-being.

In addition to cardiovascular exercise—which accelerates the heart rate and builds endurance—there are other forms of exercise that can help rid your body of toxins, such as yoga, which focuses on deep stretching, increasing circulation, posture, and balance. Let's look at the variety of exercises you can enjoy to enhance and complement your detox experience.

RAWESOME TIP

Do your chores! Mopping the floor, scrubbing your bathroom, and outdoor chores like raking and mowing count as exercise and are good for your health.

Yoga

You may be familiar with yoga as a gentle exercise practice that involves specific postures and movements that stretch, twist, and bend the body. The yoga exercises done at health centers and yoga studios all stem from a tradition that is several thousands of years old. These traditions have their origins in India, going back as early as 1700 B.C.E. The ancient practice of yoga encompassed a disciplined practice where control of the body led to control of the mind—and eventually, to a supreme contemplative state. Control over the body is a good start for many, while advanced yoga practitioners also explore breathing exercises, meditation, and cleansing procedures.

The physical postures in yoga are called asanas. Each posture is specifically designed to stimulate a response in the body and cultivate a deeper discipline in the mind. The postures in yoga are practiced in a progressive series, which allow them to build upon each other. There are a variety of postures, ranging from balancing, stretching, inversions, and meditative poses.

In its simplest form, yoga represents a low-impact form of exercise that assists with body detox. In a more holistic form, yoga represents a practice that cultivates mind, body, and spirit. For the raw food detox program, yoga serves a specific purpose of stretching and moving all parts of the body, thus increasing circulation and blood flow. Parts of the body are completely neglected throughout the course of the average workday, and yoga gives some much-needed attention to those areas—a gentle stretch and a fresh supply of oxygen-rich blood.

Many yoga postures massage the internal organs of the body as well, allowing fresh, oxygen-rich blood to flow in while stagnant blood is moved out. This is great for detox and particularly for digestion. Circulation, respiration, oxygenation, detoxification, and relaxation all combine to make yoga an integral part of your raw food detox and can help make your program more successful.

Rebounding

Who would have thought that when you were jumping on the bed as a kid that you had stumbled upon one of the most effective and simplest forms of healing exercise? Rebounding is a form of exercise that uses a mini-trampoline, which enables the user to bounce repeatedly. A rebounding trampoline is designed specifically for low-impact and low-altitude bouncing. Rebounding employs the forces of acceleration, deceleration, and gravity to provide exercise for every cell in the body with an equal amount of force. Rebounding is unique in that it gets the intracellular fluid known as lymph circulating.

Most other forms of cardiovascular exercise employ resistance from friction and forward movement. Rebounding harnesses the force of gravity and the up-and-down motion provided by the rebounding device. The beauty of rebounding is that once you have a quality rebounding device, you can use it practically anywhere—and it's suitable for use by almost everyone. When it's cold or raining, you can rebound inside. When it's sunny, put the rebounder on your outside deck and exercise in the sun. In the book *Jumping for Health* by Dr. Morton Walker, the numerous benefits and testimonials from rebound users highlight health and healing potential provided by this simple device. The book even offers illustrations of the multiple ways a person can exercise, including therapeutic techniques for the elderly or disabled individuals.

Some of the benefits of rebounding include:

- Increased lung capacity
- Oxygenation of the entire body
- Increased red blood cell count
- Opening and increased function of capillaries
- Improved respiration
- Optimization of heart rate
- Lowering of *LDL* and raising of *HDL* levels in the blood
- Blood thinning
- Enhanced metabolism

- Improved digestion
- Improved elimination
- Aerobic conditioning
- Muscle toning
- Weight loss

DEFINITION

LDL (low-density lipoprotein) is the bad type of cholesterol that can contribute to heart disease.

HDL (high-density lipoprotein) is the good type of cholesterol that can protect against heart disease.

Cardio and Sweating

"Getting your cardio" seems to be a common battle cry for the athletically inclined, but what does that actually mean? "Cardio" is short for cardiovascular exercise, which is all about the heart, circulation, and the exchange of oxygen and carbon dioxide in the blood. Lung capacity and respiratory efficiency figures into the cardio equation, because that's where the blood gets its oxygen and eliminates its CO_2.

Cardio is any exercise that increases the heart rate for a sustained period of time with a specific intensity. Oxygen intake and usage in cellular respiration is central to cardiovascular exercise (also referred to as aerobic exercise), which includes bicycling, running, swimming, and walking. Jumping rope is one of the most efficient ways to get your aerobic exercise, as is jogging—but both of these forms are jarring (high impact) on the knees and hips. If joint issues are a problem for you, it may be best to choose another cardio form. Interestingly, the best form of low-impact aerobic exercise that combines the benefits of both jogging and skipping rope is rebounding.

When you exercise, especially when you do aerobic exercise, you sweat—and when you sweat, you help purge toxins from the body. Sweating is both a cooling and eliminative process. During and after exercise, it is necessary to replace water and electrolytes in the body. Processed, high-sugar "sports drinks" are not the proper route for rehydrating and remineralizing the body. What the body needs is simple, whole-food sugars, organic minerals, and pure water. The best source of these is fresh fruit and vegetable juices. Coconut water is also another source of electrolyte-rich hydration. Fresh fruit is an easy way to replenish the body's minerals and hydration. Water-rich citrus fruits or melons make for a great post-workout meal, particularly during your detoxification program.

> **DETOXER'S ALERT**
>
> As with all types of exercise, and in particular when doing cardiovascular exercise, be sure that your doctor approves of its nature and intensity, especially if you suffer from any specific conditions or illnesses. If you are not used to much exercise of any type, go slowly and do as much as is comfortable while you are detoxing.

Outside Assistance

The key to an effective and healthy detox program is not only in the food—it's in multiple forms of detox support. While hydrating whole foods and pure water take care of your insides, a number of external methods are supportive of cleansing. Once again, we can use the car analogy in which fuel/food is only one aspect of a properly functioning and good-looking ride. The "outside" support systems for your detox program are like taking your car to get detailed. They complement the "inner" work you've begun with the raw foods and add to your healthy glow.

Skin Brushing

People brush their teeth and hair, but they rarely brush their skin. Remember that inch for inch, the skin is the body's largest eliminative organ and a visible indicator of internal health. In the course of a day, the skin can eliminate up to two pounds of toxins. Dry skin can signal dehydration while oily skin can be an indicator of a sluggish liver. Pale skin may indicate that you need to get some sun, and flabby skin may indicate a need for exercise. One simple way to give some love to your skin is by engaging in dry skin brushing every morning. Dry skin brushing is different than scrubbing yourself in the shower in that no water is involved and a medium- or hard-bristled vegetable-fiber brush is used. Skin brushing removes dead skin particles and toxins that have been pushed out through the pores. It helps stimulate blood circulation and the growth of new skin.

You'll need to purchase a handled soft brush designed specifically for dry skin brushing. You can find these brushes at health stores or online. The procedure for dry skin brushing starts by shedding your clothes and then vigorously brushing your body. Start with the bottoms of your feet. Work your way up the legs to your buttocks. Give your thighs a healthy brushing. Once you're at the waist area, brush the palms of your hands and work toward the chest, working from the extremities toward the heart. Lightly brush the stomach and chest, and finish with the back. The skin of the face is too sensitive for skin brushing and is best cleansed and exfoliated with gentler methods, such as a soft soap-free washcloth in the shower.

Massage

Massage is a wonderful way to encourage the elimination of toxins through the skin. There are a variety of massage methods, each with its own specific benefits, but in general, all massage stimulates circulation, encourages detox, softens and breaks up mineral deposits and scar tissue, reduces cellulite, and aids in relaxation. A quality massage is so effective in eliminating toxins that it's highly recommended to consume several glasses of water after receiving a massage to maintain hydration and help remove loosened toxins. Massage is a powerful ally during fasting as well because of its role in supporting the body's detoxification process.

Saunas and Steam

Saunas and steam baths both use heat to achieve their purpose. The main difference between the two is whether the heat is dry (sauna) or moist (steam bath). Both sauna and steam achieve their detoxing power through sweating caused by heat. The moist heat of the steam bath can soften and soothe the skin and moisten the lungs. This is beneficial, though, only if the sauna is chlorine free. Some steam rooms use herbal blends that soothe the lungs and are excellent for respiratory conditions. Both the steam and sauna are beneficial for detoxification because they encourage circulation, revitalize the skin, and relax the musculatory system.

A newer type of sauna known as the Far Infrared Sauna (FIR) has been shown to be particularly good at aiding detoxification. The FIR sauna is a step up from the regular sauna that uses only a heating coil to warm things up. FIR saunas use a spectrum of light that is just past infrared in its wavelength. Far infrared light has been identified as naturally occurring when the sun is lowest on the horizon at sunrise and sunset. During the rest of the day, it is overpowered by ultraviolet and infrared light. Far infrared light has been shown to have a healing effect because it is able to penetrate the body.

Although we can't see infrared light, we feel it when we step out into the sun or touch the skin of a warm-blooded creature. The wavelength of infrared light determines the level at which it can penetrate an object before it begins to vibrate its cells. This is how far infrared is employed in detoxification. In a FIR sauna, there is both infrared radiation (surface heat) and far infrared (subsurface heat) heating working in tandem. So, the standard heating element heats you from the outside—causing you to sweat—while the far infrared light penetrates the skin, vibrates the cells, and facilitates detox from within.

FRESH FACT

FIR saunas have been shown to be highly effective in detoxing individuals who have substance abuse problems. In drug and alcohol rehabilitation, withdrawal symptoms are often the biggest challenge—and these types of saunas can expedite the process of detoxification and simultaneously reduce withdrawal symptoms.

You don't need a FIR sauna to take advantage of the healing benefits of far infrared light, however. Products of all shapes, sizes, and prices have been developed that use far infrared technology. Heating pads, massage devices, and far infrared lamps are just a few of the consumer options. Many health facilities have added FIR saunas to part of their healing and treatment programs. The Internet has a wealth of information about far infrared as well as products available for consumers.

Acupuncture

Eastern medicine has known for centuries about the healing benefits of acupuncture. It is only recently that this ancient art of healing has begun to gain acceptance. In study after study, acupuncture has shown positive results in relieving pain and many other health conditions. The World Health Organization (WHO) and United States National Institute of Health (NIH) have both acknowledged acupuncture as effective in treating pain and neurological conditions.

Traditional Chinese medicine employs acupuncture in balancing the energies—the yin and yang—of the body. The central idea in acupuncture regards the energy pathways in the body known as meridians. The practitioner uses needles or other forms of stimulation to move and balance energy along these pathways.

The role of acupuncture in detox is supportive in balancing energy in the systems of elimination. Acupuncture can be effective in moving stuck energy in stagnant areas of the body. Once energy gets moving, toxins are often released—beginning a healthy cycle of cleansing. Search online or inquire at a holistic physician's office to find a trained acupuncture therapist in your area.

> **FRESH FACT**
>
> Sound has been successfully used in moving stuck energy in the body. This method of acupuncture is known as acutonics and can provide pain relief and accelerated healing from injuries when employed with traditional Chinese medicine.

Inside Assistance

Food as medicine is at the heart of raw food detox, yet sometimes you need to bring some specialty non-food items into the edible equation to provide some healing support. As strange as it may seem, these substances are primarily inert compounds that pass through the body unabsorbed while others can be nutrient-dense and mineral-rich foods. What they all will provide, however, is the ability to bind to toxins and assist in carrying them out of the body. Let's meet some of these detoxification allies.

Clays

Edible clays have been part of healing traditions around the world, practiced by tribes in the Andes, Central Africa, and in Australia. Animals have also been observed consuming certain types of clay. Research has shown that some clays, specifically montmorillonite, have some curious healing properties. Montmorillonite clay is named for the region of France in which it was discovered.

The same type of clay has since been discovered in other parts of the world, including Fort Benton, Wyoming, for which bentonite clay is named. Bentonite, which is actually a volcanic ash, is a common ingredient in many cleansing products because of its capability to pass through the body while binding to harmful toxins and effortlessly removing them. When bentonite clay is mixed with water, its surface area expands—allowing it to absorb up to 40 times its weight in toxins. It is a negatively charged solution that naturally binds with positively charged toxins, bacteria, and viruses.

Consuming bentonite clay has also been shown effective in cases of food poisoning and heavy metal poisoning. When used in conjunction with fasting, it can help alleviate detox symptoms by removing toxins from the intestines.

Bentonite should never be consumed in a dry form. It is best when mixed with water and a bulking agent, such as chia seeds or psyllium husk powder, to make a cleansing shake. Be sure to read the instructions on the container and follow the recommended frequency.

This combination passes through the digestive system and soaks up toxins along the way, eventually being eliminated from the bowels. Bentonite clay in liquid form can be used topically as well to treat insect stings and bites, pimples, and boils.

Zeolite

Zeolites are a mineral class that's volcanic in origin. The unique characteristic of zeolite minerals is their crystalline structure and negative charge. Zeolite works in a similar way to bentonite in that it binds to toxins and escorts them from the body.

Zeolite products aren't confined in their use for the digestive tract, however. Many zeolite solutions are fine enough to pass through the blood-brain barrier and aid in detoxing all parts of the body. Once zeolite has bound itself to toxins and neutralized its charge, it exits the body through urine or feces. Zeolite has been shown to be effective in removing heavy metals and toxins from the body while also supporting immune function. Typically, zeolite supplements are taken in liquid form by adding them to water, smoothies, or juices. There are also zeolite capsules, which can be swallowed.

The Internet is overloaded with different zeolite products these days. This wasn't the case a few years ago. Zeolite has many uses in a variety of industries, so there are many different grades of zeolite. It's difficult to know whether you are getting a quality product or low-grade rock dust, so look for Waiora Natural Cellular Defense and Super-Z-Lite from Omica Organics, which are highly reputable. Both can easily found online. Follow the accompanying directions regarding preparation and frequency.

Fulvic Acid

An organic electrolyte that is a natural compound occurring in living soils and living plants, fulvic acid has been shown to have a rejuvenating effect on living cells. Fulvic acid has been extensively used in farming for decades and is now gaining attention for its role as an animal and human supplement. Research has shown fulvic acid to be effective in successful grafting and transplant acceptance in animals as well as eliminating infection, increasing nutrient absorption, and removing parasites. Follow the directions on the packaging for preparation and frequency.

Sea Veggies

Sea vegetables are often referred to as "sea weeds," which is quite an injustice considering their food value and healing potential. These plants are resourceful, resilient, and hardy, not to mention nutrient dense. Sea vegetables are a class of food that grows wild along ocean shorelines and in inland waterways. They can be either saltwater or freshwater, although saltwater types are the most commonly found.

The mineral-rich medium in which sea vegetables grow bestows upon them a dynamic array of vitamins and minerals. When compared to land-based crops, seaweed has 10 to 20 times more minerals. Each of the major sea veggies has particular specialized nutrients. For example, wakame is higher in omega-3 fatty acids than other sea vegetables, while laver is high in vitamin A. All the sea vegetables rank high for optimal health support and weight loss as well.

Sea vegetables are a natural source of iodine, a vital nutrient important for proper thyroid function. The sea vegetable kelp contains high amounts of organic iodine and can be used as a dietary source of iodine. Individuals who have elevated iodine levels or a thyroid condition should consult their healthcare practitioner before incorporating sea vegetables into their diet, however.

Seaweed excels in detoxing the body of heavy metals and radioactive toxins. They contain alginic acid, which binds to these toxins and escorts them out. Sea veggies are also alkalizing and antimicrobial and can be easily incorporated into soups, sauces, and salads in your raw food detox program.

Water Flow and Waste

Water (consumed) hydrates the cells of the body and assists in the elimination of toxins. The act of drinking water, however, is not the only method for taking water into the body. Washing the exterior of the body removes dead skin and toxins and invigorates the cells, and this is something most of us do on a regular basis. But there is another very effective way that uses water to remove massive amounts of toxins from the bowels: colon hydrotherapy.

Colon Hydrotherapy

Simply put, colon hydrotherapy is the therapeutic use of water to clean the colon. This practice is nothing new; ancient cultures such as the Egyptians and Romans practiced forms of colon hydrotherapy, also called irrigation. Hippocrates, the "Father of Medicine," employed the use of water in the colon for healing as well. In fact, colon hydrotherapy was considered a staple in early modern medical practices, and colon irrigation machines were common in hospitals and doctors' offices until the 1930s, when alternative practices for digestive conditions were often traded for more intrusive treatments such as surgery.

Currently, there has been a reemergence of colon hydrotherapy in holistic healing practices. While part of the medical establishment chooses to dismiss the historical and popular modern-day use of colon hydrotherapy, testimonials and dramatic accounts of healing continue today.

If you would like to supplement your raw food detoxification program with colon hydrotherapy, you will probably find it to be a significant and helpful approach to toxin removal. Cleanses and enemas are the easiest and lowest on the technical scale for home hydrotherapy, and there is abundant information in books and online to guide you through the process.

FRESH FACT

Dr. John H. Kellogg operated a health resort in Battle Creek, Michigan, where he specialized in treating gastrointestinal disorders in the early 1900s. In his practice, he treated more than 40,000 patients using colon hydrotherapy and reported a 90 percent success rate in which only 20 patients required surgery for bowel dysfunction. He documented these astounding results in the *American Journal of Medicine* in 1917.

Cleanses and Enemas

The purpose behind colon cleansing with water is to flush toxic debris out of the colon using water. A person who has a normally functioning bowel who has spent a lifetime eating natural foods in proper amounts, drinking pure water, and living in a pristine environment probably has no need for such a procedure. Unfortunately, it's safe to say that most of us are not in this category. The results of our daily living in a world of convenience, excess, and toxins is toxic sludge, often referred to as mucoid plaque.

Why would the body hold onto this toxic sludge? Well, why do you have stacks of old newspapers in your garage or basement or some past-their-prime vegetables and leftovers hiding in the back of your refrigerator? Overwork and neglect are two of the reasons, and at least for the body, another is self-preservation. Remember, the body will wrap toxins in mucus as well as fat to protect itself, and these toxic accumulations are not easily eliminated because of their lack of fiber (among other things). Flushing the colon with water helps remove this toxic debris and prevent it from being reabsorbed.

Colon irrigation can be super low-tech or more involved, requiring a trained technician. There are three basic items needed (not including water): a tip, a tube, and a container. You can buy the needed equipment online or at a pharmacy. Just look for an enema kit, hot water bag, or douche bag. All you have to supply is pure water. The water used, however, is of major importance. Tap water is absolutely unacceptable for use in colon irrigation unless it has been filtered and purified. Distilled water is the best choice for internal flushing.

Enemas are effective at alleviating constipation, headaches, and bloating, but they prove themselves indispensable for a cleansing and fasting program. It is best to perform an enema after you have had a regular bowel movement. If you have chronic constipation, any time is a good time. Warm water should be used (just below or at body temperature works well).

Enemas do have limitations, though. The entire length of the colon is around five feet long, and the volume of water in an enema and the method of delivery doesn't get very deep into the bowels. A specialist known as a colon hydrotherapist has the equipment and training that allow for a deeper and more thorough internal cleansing. These therapists can clean the entire length of the colon using a procedure called a colonic. Once extensive colon cleansing has taken place and a healthy diet has been established, colonics can be taken seasonally or during fasting periods.

FRESH FACT

Dr. Max Gerson (1881–1959) developed the use of the coffee enema over the course of his healing practice, during which he treated many patients successfully who were deemed terminal. He highlights some of his successes in his book *A Cancer Therapy: A Result of 50 Cases*. He is one of the pioneers who led to the renaissance of natural healing and colon hydrotherapy.

Implants and Suppositories

Implants are a method of injecting a specific liquid into the colon for healing and cleansing purposes. The same type of plastic tip used for enemas is often used for implants. The enema bag may be used, but a large-volume syringe also works well. The amount of liquid in an implant is only a few ounces and is supposed to be retained in the colon until a regular bowel movement occurs. Implants are often taken before bed and allowed to remain in the colon overnight. Probiotics and wheatgrass juice are some of the items often used for implants.

Suppositories are solid capsules inserted into the rectum. They are usually composed of a material such as cacao butter that will dissolve after it is inserted into the body. Suppositories are meant to release a specific substance over time. Glycerin suppositories are a common natural remedy for constipation. They release glycerin into the bowel and aid in elimination. For cleansing and detox, there are a variety of suppositories that contain compounds that are meant to detox heavy metals and toxins from the colon.

If you would like to incorporate implants or suppositories into the raw food detoxification program, be sure to consult your physician and always follow the directions for preparation and frequency on the product label.

The Least You Need to Know

- Exercise, whether cardio, aerobic, or low-impact stretching and yoga, can stimulate digestive activity and cleansing.
- Attending to the outside of the body with practices such as skin brushing, massage, and heat through sauna or steam can help remove toxins.
- Colon hydrotherapy has been practiced for centuries and can prove valuable in eliminating toxins.
- When used in conjunction with raw food detox, colon-cleansing methods are maximized and detox symptoms are minimized.

Getting Started

Here, we'll delve into the nitty-gritty of the program. Starting with a scorecard for you to determine which plan you should begin with, we'll then look at the individual programs in detail and see the actual menus and foods you'll be enjoying.

In this part, you'll also get help setting up your kitchen for the program with helpful equipment and paraphernalia that will assist you in preparing all the terrific recipes. Finally, we'll touch on some social challenges you may face during your raw food detoxification program and how to cope with them and gain as much support from family and friends as you can.

Where to Begin?

In This Chapter

- The Raw Food Detox Score Card
- Important factors for evaluating where to start
- Detox Programs A, B, C, and D—a quick review

It's time to take the plunge and get started! But where to begin? Before you know how far you need to go toward improving your health, you need to figure out exactly where you are—and the Raw Food Detox Score Card will help you do that. Whether you have lots of weight to lose and numerous poor eating habits to change or are close to a desirable weight but want to look and feel more lively and vibrant, the score card assessment will evaluate your needs and pinpoint the program level you should use as your detox starting point.

Several important factors will influence the score you receive, and the amount of weight you wish to lose is only one part of the evaluation. You'll also be answering questions about your bowel regularity, medications you are taking, and the types of foods you are currently consuming (from processed to organics). The amount of exercise you do is also an important component.

Jot down your answers to the upcoming questions and score accordingly. Once the tally is in, you'll be able to preview the program level you'll be starting with. A brief description of what you need to accomplish as well as the terrific improvements you'll discover will be outlined for each program, from A to D. Then, in the next chapter, you'll take a look at the terrific menus you can look forward to. Before you know it, you'll be on your way to a dynamic detoxification and a healthier and happier you.

Raw Detox Score Card

The Raw Food Detox Score Card will help you determine where to begin your detox plan. The seven different categories serve as a guide to gauging your present health situation. However, once you start your personalized program, these numbers will naturally begin to change.

For example, weight loss may occur within the first week, while regularity can increase as well. And once you've stocked your cupboards and refrigerator with more raw, whole, and chemical-free foods, the next three categories regarding toxins, cooked versus raw, and organic versus regular will change, too.

Last but not least, as you begin to feel livelier and healthier, you'll want to increase the amount of time you dedicate to exercise—following the recommendations set in Chapter 4—and consequently, these numbers will change as well. For now, however, rate yourself according to where you are at this moment in time in all these categories. After a week or two, consider retaking the score card test and adjusting your program as desired.

Here's what the quick reference card looks like. Let's take a look at each category in a little more depth.

Weight Goals	Number of Medications	Regularity	Food Toxins	Cooked versus Raw	Organic versus Conventional	Exercise: Days Per Week	Score
0 or gain weight	0	3/3	0–1	80–90%	75–100%	4+	0
Lose 5–15	1	3/2	1–2	70–80%	50–75%	2–3	1
Lose 15–30	2	3/1	2–3	60–70%	25–50%	1–2	2
Lose 30+	3	3/0	3–4	50–60%	0–25%	0	3

Total Points	Program Level
17+	*Program A for "Achievement"*
10–16	*Program B for "Best Foods"*
5–9	*Program C for "Commitment"*
1–4	*Program D for "Discipline"*

Weight Goals

This is the number of pounds you want to lose, which is often the primary focus for many detoxers. Weight loss is usually easy with a raw foods diet. As the body purges toxins, it naturally sheds weight. The first column represents the amount of weight you want to lose. The more weight you want to lose, the more detox you may experience and the more important it is to take your time with the raw food detox program. Rapid weight loss usually means rapid detox, which may be uncomfortable. Raw food detox should be an enjoyable experience for the most part. There will be some "speed bumps" along the way, but all in all it should be a most enjoyable ride.

- If you don't want to lose weight: 0 points
- If you want to lose 5 to 15 pounds: 1 point
- If you want to lose 15 to 30 pounds: 2 points
- If you want to lose more than 30 pounds: 3 points

Medications

The "Number of Medications" column lists the number of medications you are currently taking. Remember that if you are regularly taking medication of any kind (prescribed or over-the-counter), you should consult your healthcare practitioner regarding whether a raw food detox is right for you. Do not include vitamins and supplements when figuring out your score. In many cases, medication needs will be reduced and possibly eliminated after successfully completing the raw food detox program. Be sure to monitor your progress and check in with your doctor along the way.

- If you take no medications: 0 points
- If you take one medication: 1 point
- If you take two medications: 2 points
- If you take three or more medications: 3 points

DETOXER'S ALERT

Certain medications, such as those taken to control high blood pressure and thin the blood, carry warnings of consuming dark-green, leafy vegetables (such as spinach and kale) due to their effect on vitamin K levels and blood clotting. Be sure to ask your doctor about this issue if you take high blood pressure medicine.

Regularity

The "Regularity" column represents how many bowel movements you have a day in relation to how many meals you eat. As discussed before, ideally you should be having as many movements as you have meals per day. For example, if you eat two meals a day and have two movements, then there is little room for improvement in this category and your score would be zero.

Most of us are not as prolific, however, when it comes to bathroom habits—especially those whose detox needs are great.

If you are moving your bowels every other day but regularly eating three meals a day, then you would select "3/0" (three meals—zero movements) and score three points. If you eat more than three meals a day, just take into account the number of movements you have a day and score accordingly with 3 as the maximum number of meals.

- If you have three movements after three meals: 0 points
- If you have two movements after three meals: 1 point
- If you have one movement after three meals: 2 points
- If you are irregular or skip a day: 3 points

Food Toxins

This category refers to processed foods, and it is likely that most people—except for the healthiest of us—will score high. That's because processed foods, or "food toxins" (as raw foodists prefer to call them), are all products that contain the following common ingredients:

- White sugar and/or corn syrup
- White flour
- White rice and potatoes
- *Trans fats* and/or chemical food additives

DEFINITION

Trans fats, also called trans fatty acids and often designated by the term "partially hydrogenated," are unhealthy substances created during the heating of oils in cooking and have been linked to heart disease, obesity, and diabetes.

For scoring purposes, select the number of servings of these items you consume in a day. This includes processed snacks, chips, breads, pastries, and fried foods. For example, if you regularly consume a bagel and a café latte for breakfast and a hamburger and fries at lunch, you have already hit the four servings mark (and that's just half your day!). Be honest in this category, and know that this may be the toughest nut to crack in your detox program. With all the new tasty alternatives offered in the upcoming recipe section, however, it should be easy to switch out these harmful foods with some delicious and healthy alternatives.

- One or fewer servings per day: 0 points
- No more than two servings per day: 1 point
- No more than three servings per day: 2 points
- Four or more servings per day: 3 points

Cooked Versus Raw

For this category, you'll need to figure an average percentage of how much raw food you eat in a day as opposed to food that has been cooked (estimate by volume and not by calories). Although it may seem at first to be a tough prospect eating even just 70 percent raw, chances are you'll make great strides in this category early on. Because breakfast really sets the tone for the day, if you start with fruits and juices (as you'll be doing in the program), this will allow you to taper your eating toward more complex foods at dinnertime—even including a good amount of cooked selections. Before you know it, your raw percentage will be up and your overall score will be down.

- If 80 to 90 percent of your diet is raw: 0 points
- If 70 to 80 percent of your diet is raw: 1 point
- If 60 to 70 percent of your diet is raw: 2 points
- If less than 60 percent of your diet is raw: 3 points

Organic Versus Conventional

This category can highlight two aspects of your present health and detoxification requirements. First, it is a gauge of the toxic load you may be taking in by eating conventionally grown produce. Because pesticides and chemical growth enhancers are commonly used in traditional farming, this adds to your toxic load. How much organically grown food you are eating is also an indicator of the nutrient content you're likely getting from what you eat, because fewer vitamins and minerals are leeched out through chemical contamination. Organic foods tend to pack a more powerful punch nutritionally—particularly in the antioxidant department. Locally grown, chemical-free foods can also be included on the organic side, along with anything grown in your organic home garden.

Don't forget the many packaged organic foods that are also available and which you may be consuming already, such as cereals, nuts, and grains. If you're not already, you'll want to take advantage of the vast array of organic whole-food snacking options available at health food and grocery stores. The goal is to eliminate the consumption of foods contaminated with toxins as well as increase nutrition. When you bring your "organic" percentage up, you'll experience a definite difference in health:

- If 75 to 100 percent of your diet is organic: 0 points

- If 50 to 75 percent of your diet is organic: 1 point

- If 25 to 50 percent of your diet is organic: 2 points

- If less than 25 percent of your diet is organic: 3 points

RAWESOME TIP

When reading food packaging, be sure to check the ingredient list as well as the front to discern whether all the ingredients contained in the product are indeed organically produced. If unclear, contact the company to know for sure.

Exercise

This category represents how active you are on a weekly basis. Exercise doesn't need to be a one- to two-hour session at the gym. It can be a 30-minute bike ride, yoga in the morning, or a brisk walk in the neighborhood. Being physically active helps melt fat away, removes toxins from the body, and increases aerobic capacity. A little exercise goes a long way, so it's worthwhile to make it part of your daily routine.

Ideally, if we all could do four days a week of rebounding (see Chapter 4 for more about rebounding), global health statistics would dramatically change. If you don't have a rebounder, then just gently dance to your favorite music. The idea is to get your blood circulating and your heart rate elevated for at least 10 minutes. Make a playlist of 10 of your favorite songs, and you're likely to have an enjoyable half-hour workout.

- If you exercise four or more days per week: 0 points
- If you exercise two or three days per week: 1 point
- If you exercise one or two days per week: 2 points
- If you do little or no exercise: 3 points

Determine Your Score

Figure out your personal score by adding the results for each category. If you're on the border of one of the programs, use your discretion in choosing which program you wish to follow. Choosing program A over B will be an easier way to start your program. Work your way through the raw food detox programs, staying at each level for at least a week. Your body should give you signals of whether it's time to move up to the next grade. You can update your score each week as well. When elimination catches up and weight loss stops, it may be time to move up.

Program A

If your total points came to 17 or more, you probably have a good amount of work to do. But "A" is for "achievement," and with raw food detox you will be on your way to achieving your health goals. You may be dealing with health challenges, but with discipline you can "achieve" anything. With discipline, weight and cravings will disappear. Explore all the menu options available with raw food detox and find the foods you truly enjoy. By simply increasing physical activity and the percentage of raw and chemical-free foods you eat, you can easily move up to the next program. Weight loss should happen naturally at this level—especially if you are staying hydrated and your elimination is becoming more efficient.

Program B

If you scored between 10 and 16 points, you're actually in a pretty good place but may need to make some better choices. "B" is for the "best foods" you can possibly eat. It's amazing the changes that begin to happen when you give your body what it really needs. After a week or two at this level, you may want to get your blood pressure and cholesterol levels checked if you had issues. You may be pleasantly surprised at the results. Follow your physician's instructions regarding any medication you may have been taking. As your regularity improves and as you lose weight, be sure to recalculate your score. Program "C" is within your reach.

Program C

"C" is for "commitment," and if your score is between five and nine points, this is why you have made it this far. "Commitment" is the point where discipline forms and you begin to see the fruits of your labor. At this stage, your regularity should have improved while weight-loss goals are close to being met. Many physical conditions have been alleviated. Improvements should also be seen in physical stamina and mental clarity. You may often find yourself "in the zone" while working and working out. Keep enjoying a high percentage of raw and chemical-free foods while remaining active as you push toward program D.

Program D

"D" is for the "discipline" that you have cultivated to make it this far, and if your score is four points or fewer, you've reached the top of the mountain. How do you like the view? Stay at the D level until you've achieved all your health goals. After two weeks of the D program, you should be able to determine what you want to do next. If you wish to experience deeper cleansing, consider doing some of the juicing, fasting, or cleansing protocols listed in the book. Now that you have achieved a higher level of health, look at the Raw Detox Score Card and see which areas don't even apply to you anymore. It's amazing what you can *achieve* with *discipline, commitment,* and the *best foods*.

The Least You Need to Know

- Using the Raw Detox Score Card will help you determine where to begin your detoxification.

- Considerations including desired weight loss, current eating and exercise habits, and any medications you take are included in the evaluation.

- Anyone regularly taking prescribed or over-the-counter medications should consult a healthcare professional before beginning the program.

- Depending on your score, you will follow raw food detox program level A, B, C, or D.

- As improvements are made, you can move up a level and increase the intensity of your raw food detoxification program.

Raw Food Detox Menus

Chapter 6

In This Chapter

- Important practices for all levels
- Specific menus for each level of detox
- Possible cleansing reactions

As you get ready to plunge into your detoxification, you are probably wondering what's on the menu. For each program level from A to D, you'll find a comprehensive recommended menu that draws from the recipes in this book. But there are also a few points that are valid for every level, and we'll take a look at those first so you are sure to include these rituals as part of your program.

Depending on your score from the last chapter and how ambitious you are to dive into your detoxification, you'll be following one of the four menu plans in this chapter. You can always re-evaluate yourself on the scorecard if you feel ready to make a move up to a more challenging level. Do try to stick with each level for at least a week or two before changing.

As you begin detoxing, you will probably notice several symptoms occurring in the way you feel and the way your body reacts to raw food. These normal reactions are outlined at the end of this chapter so you will have a good idea of what to expect as you begin the process of detoxification.

About the Programs

Now that you have determined your raw food detox score, let's take a look at the menus. If you have some other raw food recipe books or raw food recipe favorites, feel free to rotate them into the program, as the menus listed are only suggestions.

Programs A and B start with 15 days of recipes, with several repeating throughout the week. Programs C and D are simple seven-day plans that can easily be repeated. It's a good idea to test some of the recipes ahead of time as you prepare yourself for the detox diet. That way, you'll know which ones you may wish to avoid and those that may become favorites (which will help you in your shopping). However, there are some recipes that should be part of your daily routine. Try to get in at least one soup and/or smoothie a day—and if you are juicing, try for at least one of those as well. By the time you get to program D, you will be enjoying mostly soups, juices, and smoothies all day long.

As you move through the programs, be sure to transition gradually. Jumping from program A to program D is not recommended because it may cause a rapid detox. It is also recommended, when ending the detox program, that you slowly transition from program D to eating more solid and complex foods over the course of at least a week. This will allow your digestion and elimination time to adjust to the foods that weren't part of your detox program.

 RAWESOME TIP

Greens are nutrient dense, light on calories, and quick exiting, so be sure to have some fruit or juice 20 minutes before your main meal.

Morning Ritual

Begin every day, regardless of your program level, with a 16-ounce glass of purified water and a squirt of fresh lemon juice. Add a pinch of sea salt or Himalayan salt if you like. If you want it warm, heat the water on the stove top (no microwaving) or in a kettle.

To effectively detox, you will need to abstain from drinking coffee—a morning ritual you may have been accustomed to. If this is a difficult prospect at first, consider drinking one of the following substitutes after your lemon water:

- Green tea (decaffeinated and organic)

- Yerba Maté (tea made from a South American shrub)

- Teechino (an herbal caffeine-free coffee)

- Genmaicha (brown rice tea from Japan)

- Pero (a grain-based coffee substitute)

Evening Ritual

One to two hours before bedtime drink a 16-ounce glass of purified water. Give your-self enough time before bed so you won't have to run to the bathroom during the night. Hydration is critical while you are detoxing and so is sleep. Alcohol, coffee, sweetened sodas, and artificially sweetened drinks all dehydrate the body. Only pure water and the water in fresh fruits, young coconuts, and vegetables are truly hydrat-ing for the body.

Keep the Order

Eat the foods for each meal in the order they are listed. The parentheses with a num-ber inside indicate the suggested time you should wait before eating the next food item. For example, "(20)" means wait 20 minutes before you eat the next food. Be sure to refer to Chapter 3 and Appendix B when necessary for food-combining tips.

RAWESOME TIP

If you have to go out to eat, you can pack a dressing and order a large salad. If you have to attend a family event, put together a hearty raw dish that will keep you satisfied and fend off temptation. Some travel-friendly staples are apples, avocados, nuts, seeds, and dried fruit.

Watch Your Portions

When you start the program, your perspective on portion size may be skewed—especially if you have been primarily eating nutrient-deficient foods. Surprisingly, a little may end up going a long way. By all means, start by preparing serving sizes that you think will satisfy you, but be aware of the amount that actually satisfies you. There should be a difference. Many people look at a raw food meal and say to themselves, "That's not going to be enough." Often at the end of the meal, though, there's food left on the plate. As you progress through the menus, portion sizes should naturally decrease. Remember, you are getting high-quality nutrition. There's no need to pile on the food like you did back when it was nutrient deficient and you were constantly hungry.

Eat Dessert

Don't think that we forgot desserts on this menu. As far as I am concerned, you can have dessert in place of or after every meal! However, eat only until you are satisfied. There are a variety of premade raw desserts available in stores, such as raw chocolate bars, pies, macaroons, brownies, cookies, and ice cream. There are also a number of raw dessert recipes included in the recipe section. If your dessert is complex, it can be eaten after your meal. Fruit is a different story, though. Because fruit is fast digesting and we're trying to avoid digestive traffic jams, you should wait at least two hours after your meal before you eat fresh fruit.

Program A: 15 Days—Easy Does It

Here's the simplest form of the program and the one that is best for those who scored rather high on their evaluation and have a lot of work to do as far as detoxification is concerned. With a good amount of cooked selections in the evening, raw food will make up approximately two thirds of your diet—still a challenge for many who are not used to the change. Stick with it, and each day will naturally become easier.

Program A Menu

Day	Morning	Midday	Snack	Evening
1	Fruit, 1–2 pieces (20), *Morning Slice*	*Lettuce Wraps* and flax crackers	*Monkey King* or other smoothie	Large green salad with *Almond Miso Sauce*, *Veggie Pizza*
2	Raw granola with *Easy Almond Mylk* or *Hemp Mylk*	Large green salad and *Almond Miso Sauce*, flax crackers	Carrot and celery slices with *Cashew Cheeze*	Large green salad with dressing, *Baked Spaghetti* or *Acorn Squash* with *Cheezy Sauce*

Day	Morning	Midday	Snack	Evening
3	*Hemp Seed Supreme Smoothie*	*Eggless Egg Salad* on sprouted bread	Raw snack bar or a few pieces of fruit	Large green salad with dressing, quinoa pasta, and *Dulse Marinara*
4	Fruit, 1–2 pieces (20), *Morning Slice*	*Sea Veggie Soup*, flax crackers	Apples with *Almond Miso Spread*	*Steamed Veggies* with *Sesame Sauce*, wild rice or sprouted bread
5	*Berry Best Smoothie*	Large green salad and *Apricot Vinaigrette*, flax crackers	*Monkey King* or other smoothie	*Massaged Kale Salad* and sprouted bread
6	Apples with *Almond Miso Spread*	*Midday Slice*	Flax crackers and *Cashew Cheeze*	*Pasta Party Kelp Noodles* with *Garlic Avo Dressing*, sprouted bread
7	*Avocado Apple Gadget*	*Lettuce Wraps*, flax crackers	Apples with *Almond Miso Spread*	Large green salad with *Almond Miso Sauce*, *Veggie Pizza*
8	Raw Granola with *Easy Almond Mylk*	*Sea Veggie Soup*, celery sticks, flax crackers	*Monkey King* or other smoothie	*Steamed Veggies* with *Sesame Sauce*, sprouted bread
9	Fruit, 1–2 pieces (20), *Morning Slice*	Large green salad and *Apricot Vinaigrette*, flax crackers	Apples with *Almond Miso Spread*	Large green salad with dressing and *Evening Slice*
10	Apples with *Almond Miso Spread*	*Tu-no Salad* on sprouted bread or sprouted wraps	Raw snack bar or a few pieces of fruit	Large green salad, quinoa pasta, marinated mushrooms, and *Dulse Marinara*
11	*Avocado Apple Gadget*	*Sea Veggie Soup*, flax crackers	Flax crackers and *Cashew Cheeze*	Large green salad with dressing, *Baked Spaghetti* or *Acorn Squash* with *Cheezy Sauce*

continues

continued

Day	Morning	Midday	Snack	Evening
12	Raw granola with *Easy Almond Mylk*	*Massaged Kale Salad* and sprouted bread	*Monkey King* or *Green Machine Smoothie*	*Steamed Veggies* with *Sesame Sauce*, wild rice or sprouted bread
13	Fruit, 1–2 pieces (20), *Morning Slice*	*Lettuce Wraps*, flax crackers	Apples with *Almond Miso Spread*	*Cauliflower Couscous* and *Evening Slice*
14	Apples with *Almond Miso Spread*	*Sea Veggie Soup*, carrot sticks, flax crackers	Raw snack bar or a few pieces of fruit	Large green salad with *Almond Miso Sauce*, *Veggie Pizza*
15	*Avocado Apple Gadget*	*Midday Slice*	Flax crackers and *Cashew Cheeze*	Large green salad, quinoa pasta, marinated mushrooms, and *Dulse Marinara*

For desserts enjoy any of the treats from Chapter 13.

Substitutions

Feel free to explore menu items on programs B, C, and D—substitutions are welcome. Most people don't change what they eat for breakfast every day of the week, although some people may enjoy exploring different recipes. I suggest looking over the menus and recipes and eventually creating your own weekly meal plan. Program A has the flexibility to incorporate all the recipes listed in the raw detox program, but as you transition into programs B through D, some cooked menu items will be replaced with simple raw items.

Raw granola and prepared snacks from the following food companies are acceptable to include during programs A and B:

- Lydia's Granola
- Two Moms in the Raw
- Go Raw
- NutsOnline.com
- Laughing Giraffe
- Kookie Karma

Program B: 15 Days—80 Percent Raw

Program B begins by introducing you to more smoothies and soups. If you compare menus A and B, you won't see any dramatic differences—but small, positive changes are being made. More and more raw food items are replacing cooked food items, and by the time you reach program D, you'll be eating all raw and mostly blended meals and juices.

Program B Menu

Day	Morning	Midday	Snack	Evening
1	*Berry Best Smoothie*	*Lettuce Wraps* and *Cucumber Dill Soup*	*Monkey King* or *Green Machine Smoothie*	Large green salad with *Almond Miso Sauce*, *Almond Pad Thai*
2	Raw granola with *Easy Almond Mylk* or *Hemp Mylk*	Large green salad and *Almond Miso Sauce*, flax crackers	Carrot and celery slices with *Cashew Cheeze*	*Cauliflower Couscous*, zucchini "noodles" with *Cheezy Sauce*
3	*Hemp Seed Supreme Smoothie*	*Midday Slice*	Raw snack bar or a few pieces of fruit	Large green salad, *Pasta Party Kelp Noodles* and *Dulse Marinara*
4	*Green Machine Smoothie*	*Sea Veggie Soup*, flax crackers	Apples with *Almond Miso Spread*	*Steamed Veggies* with *Sesame Sauce*, sprouted bread
5	*Banana Orange Kale Smoothie*	Large green salad and *Apricot Vinaigrette*, flax crackers	*Monkey King* or *Green Machine Smoothie*	*Massaged Kale Salad* and *Nori Rolls*
6	*Apple Ginger Snap Smoothie*	*Eggless Egg Salad* wrapped in cabbage leaves	Flax crackers and *Cashew Cheeze*	*Pasta Party Kelp Noodles* with *Garlic Avo Dressing*
7	*Avocado Apple Gadget*	*Lettuce Wraps* and *Sesame Curry Soup*	*Brownie Bites*	Large green salad with *Almond Miso Sauce*, *Marinated Veggies*
8	*Raw Granola* with *Easy Almond Mylk*	*Sea Veggie Soup*, celery sticks, flax crackers	*Monkey King* or *Green Machine Smoothie*	*Miso soup* and *Almond Pad Thai*

continues

continued

Day	Morning	Midday	Snack	Evening
9	1–2 pieces of fruit, (20) *Morning Slice*	Large green salad and *Apricot Vinaigrette*, flax crackers	Apples with *Almond Miso Spread*	Large green salad with dressing and *Evening Slice*
10	Apples with *Almond Miso Spread*	Carrots, celery, olives, *Cashew Cheeze*	Raw snack bar or a few pieces of fruit	Large green salad, *Pasta Party Kelp Noodles* and *Dulse Marinara*
11	*Avocado Apple Gadget*	*Sea Veggie Soup in Jar*, flax crackers	Flax crackers and *Cashew Cheeze*	Large green salad with dressing, zucchini "noodles" with *Cheezy Sauce*
12	Raw granola with *Easy Almond Mylk*	*Massaged Kale Salad* and sprouted bread	Apples with *Almond Miso Spread*	*Steamed Veggies* with *Sesame Sauce*, sprouted bread
13	*Green Machine Smoothie*	*Lettuce Wraps* and flax crackers	*Monkey King* or *Green Machine Smoothie*	*Cauliflower Couscous* and *Evening Slice*
14	Apples with *Almond Miso Spread*	*SeaVeggie Soup*, carrot sticks, flax crackers	*Superfood Truffles*	Large green salad with *Almond Miso Sauce*, *Nori Rolls*
15	*Avocado Apple Gadget*	A few pieces of fruit (20), *Tu-no Salad*	Flax crackers and *Cashew Cheeze*	Large green salad, *Pasta Party Kelp Noodles* and *Dulse Marinara*

For desserts, enjoy any of the treats from Chapter 13.

Program C: 1 to 2 Weeks—90 Percent Raw

Here, we start to separate the men from the boys (or the women from the girls). Once you've experienced a few days of program C, you should really start feeling the enormous benefits of eating this simplified diet (particularly in the energy department). Cleansing reactions may be experienced prior to elimination in the morning and possibly in the afternoon, so be sure you are calling in the reinforcements as necessary (see Chapter 4).

Program C Menu

Day	Morning	Midday	Snack	Evening
1	*Berry Best Smoothie*	*Lettuce Wraps* and *Cucumber Dill Soup*	*Monkey King* or *Green Machine Smoothie*	Large green salad with *Almond Miso Sauce*
2	*Monkey King Smoothie*	Mixed greens salad and *Almond Miso Sauce*, *Simple Miso Soup*	Carrot and celery slices with *Cashew Cheeze*	*Cauliflower Couscous*, zucchini "noodles" with *Cheezy Sauce*
3	*Hemp Seed Supreme Smoothie*	*Nori Rolls* and *Sesame Curry Soup*	Fruit (as desired)	Green salad, *Pasta Party Kelp Noodles* and *Dulse Marinara*
4	*Green Machine Smoothie*	*Sea Veggie Soup*, carrots and celery	Apples with *Almond Miso Spread*	*Stuffed Portobello* with *Sesame Sauce*
5	*Banana Orange Kale Smoothie*	Mixed greens salad and *Apricot Vinaigrette*	*Monkey King* or *Green Machine Smoothie*	*Massaged Kale Salad* and *Cucumber Dill Soup*
6	*Apple Ginger Snap Smoothie*	*Eggless Egg Salad* wrapped in cabbage leaves	Flax crackers and *Cashew Cheeze*	*Pasta Party Kelp Noodles* with *Garlic Avo Dressing*
7	*Berry Best Smoothie*	*Lettuce Wraps* and *Sesame Curry Soup*	*Brownie Bites*	Large green salad with *Almond Miso Sauce*, *Marinated Veggies*

For desserts, enjoy any of the treats from the Chapter 13.

RAWESOME TIP

When hunger hits, snack on fresh fruit or celery and carrots with tasty dips and sauces. During programs C and D, try to avoid dried snacks such as crackers or dried fruit. However, if you're really craving those snacks or are having detox challenges, go ahead and enjoy them rather than going off your detox protocol.

Program D: 1 to 2 Weeks—All Raw

If you've made it this far, give yourself a well-deserved pat on the back. While the program D menu may not be ideal for you every day of the week—and it may look a bit daunting at first—try to adhere to it as much as possible until you are finished with your detoxification and have reached most of your health goals. By now, your change in energy, weight, and overall vibrancy should be approaching remarkable.

When are you finished with the program? That is completely up to you. Take into consideration the health goals you set at the beginning when you try to decide when to finish your detox program. Who knows? You may decide to embrace a high raw food diet (75% or more) permanently (see Chapter 21).

Program D Menu

Day	Morning	Midday	Snack	Evening
1–7	Any green juice recipe with apple, carrot, or beet, and/or *Miso Soup*	Two pieces of fruit, any green juice recipe, and/or *Miso Soup*	Any green juice recipe or smoothie	Any green juice recipe and/or soup

Desserts: enjoy your choice of raw desserts at least one hour after your evening meal. With the raw food detox program, dessert isn't limited to just after dinner. Feel free to have dessert in place of meals, as a snack, or between meals. Just remember to respect food-combining rules (Chapter 3 and Appendix B), and everything should be fine. If you have blood sugar concerns, however, it may be best to abstain from too many sweet fruits and sweetened desserts. As always, consult with your healthcare provider.

Preparing Yourself

The best way to prepare yourself for your raw food detox experience is to simply continue to read. If any of the subject matter grabs your attention, then investigate it further—either on the Internet or by using the sources in the back of this book. You can also try some of the raw food recipes in advance and customize your own menu. Don't wait until you start the raw food detox program to start exercising. These are activities that can be done on a daily basis year-round. Preparing yourself also involves knowing what you can expect to experience when you embark on the raw food detox. Although they're a bit disconcerting at first, the reactions you'll have are typically good signs of healing and detoxification.

Symptoms of Healing

Cleansing reactions are integral parts of regaining your health. They are symptoms of detoxification and healing. When a person who has a long history of dietary abuses shifts to a diet of nutrient-dense, hydrating raw foods, he or she will most likely experience a cleansing reaction. Cleansing reactions are mild and short lived—the most common being loose stools, frequent bowel movements, and even diarrhea.

For someone who is chronically constipated, this may come as a shock. In fact, most people would consider healthy regularity to be abnormal because it is so uncommon and rarely experienced when on a highly processed cooked-food diet. Elimination of solids should occur within 15 to 45 minutes after consuming a meal. That's not to say that the meal you just ate is coming out of your body. This elimination should be a meal from between 15 and 24 hours prior. If you're eating three large meals a day and eliminating fewer than three times a day, technically you're constipated. So you can understand why someone new to raw foods may be alarmed when he or she ends up with a case of diarrhea or even regularity. Know that this is part of the process and nothing to be concerned about.

Other common cleansing reactions include:

- Headaches

- Body aches

- Fatigue

- A coated tongue

- Itching or rashes

- Slight fever

Reactions such as these occur when toxins are released from storage in the body at a rate that is faster than the body's ability to detox those toxins. Being that the liver is detox central in the body, the strength of your liver will determine how frequent and how strong your cleansing reactions are. As you strengthen your liver, reactions will become milder and more infrequent.

My First Cleansing Reaction

I experienced my first cleansing reaction the day I was introduced to raw foods. It was at a cleansing spa in Thailand, and I had spent all day in the kitchen learning about, preparing, and eating raw foods from the spa's resident raw food chef. I recall visiting the bathroom throughout that day of learning. That evening after a magical day of raw food fun, I began to notice a bit of fatigue, which evolved into what I call "the shakes." All I could think about was how nice it would be to go to bed, and it was only 8 P.M. I mentioned this to the very knowledgeable raw chef, and he immediately identified it as the beginning of a cleansing reaction. He reassured me that after a good night's sleep I would feel better than ever in the morning. I went to bed early that evening and experienced a mild fever and chill that kept me wrapped up in a blanket. Eventually, I drifted off to sleep and awoke the next morning feeling refreshed and symptom free. This is typical of cleansing reactions that are allowed to run their course.

The Least You Need to Know

- Whichever program level you are following, be sure to stick to the morning and evening ritual beverages.
- Menus for levels A and B provide 15 days of recipes, including a number of cooked dishes.
- Menus for levels C and D focus primarily on liquids, including soups and drinks.
- It is normal to expect certain cleansing reactions, including loose stools, fatigue, and headache.

Preparing Your Kitchen

In This Chapter

- Simple tools for basic prep
- Helpful heavy equipment
- Stocking up on raw ingredients

Gearing up your kitchen is an important step in preparing yourself for detoxification. Without the appropriate tools to assist in lightening your kitchen duties and prep, you may be reluctant to try some of the fantastic recipes to come. The harder it is to prepare your food, the less likely you'll be to give your detox plan a solid effort.

In this chapter, we take a look at the basic equipment you'll need (not too different from your average kitchen) as well as a few specialty types of tools—some heavy duty—you'll want to purchase or borrow. With a full arsenal at your disposal, you'll be more than ready to tackle even the most challenging recipe.

In addition, you'll stock up on ingredients that you'll use on a regular basis. This chapter provides a list of most items you'll need for the recipes in Part 3.

Tools of the Trade

Chances are you already have many of the basic kitchen tools. Because most of the actual "cooking" you will do involves the preparation of vegetables and fruit, you'll find that items such as frying pans and pots will become pretty obsolete while anything to do with chopping, peeling, grating, and mixing will be indispensable.

Gadgets and Knives

A good, sharp knife is a great place to start. To efficiently prepare raw foods and vegetables for juicing, it's worthwhile to invest in high-quality knives if you don't own them already. A 6- or 10-inch chef's knife and a paring knife are essential. Be sure the blade of the knife feels heavy, and avoid hollow or plastic handles.

Here are a few other gadgets to have on hand:

- Vegetable peeler
- Colanders, strainers, and sieves
- Apple corer or melon baller
- Knife sharpener and honing steel
- Measuring spoons and cups
- Rubber spatulas and wooden spoons
- Mixing bowls in various sizes
- Cutting board (preferably bamboo)
- Salad spinner
- Cheese grater
- Garlic press

 RAWESOME TIP

Although plastic or glass cutting boards are easy to clean, cutting and chopping on a wood board, particularly bamboo, is easier on both your knives and your wrist. Keep wood boards clean by washing briefly in warm, sudsy water or spray and wipe them down with distilled white vinegar diluted with water. Avoid placing wood boards in the dishwasher to ensure their longevity.

Light-Duty Equipment

The next recommended set of kitchen tools is extremely useful but not essential—especially if you are a bit of a pro in the kitchen already. However, they'll speed up your efficiency and help you make both uniform and unique cuts with ingredients.

They are not terribly expensive to purchase compared to heavy-duty equipment, so you may wish to experiment with one or two.

- Spiral slicer—This kitchen gadget enables you to cut firm fruits and vegetables into noodle shapes. This tool is ideal for making spaghetti-type recipes. Spiral slicers work well with zucchini, yellow squash, carrots, beets, radishes, sweet potatoes, apples, and more. With guidance and supervision, children can easily operate a spiral slicer and participate in preparing a healthful meal.

- Mandolin or V-slicer—This kitchen gadget has a fixed blade over which you slide fruits and vegetables to make uniform slices. The slicer has different thickness settings for creating julienne and other specialty cuts. I find these types of slicers useful when I want to quickly cut carrots, celery, and apples into a salad. There are a variety of models ranging from cheap to really expensive. I am able to do everything I need with a V-slicer costing around $30.

- Julienne peeler—This is a variation of a simple carrot/potato peeler that has multiple blades set at a perpendicular angle to the main blade, resulting in slicing long, thin strips. There are a variety of shapes and sizes available for these specialty slicers. You can often find the best selection at a local Asian market.

- Seed *mylk* bag, also known as a "paint strainer bag"—This is a very useful item that comes in a variety of shapes, sizes, and materials. The purpose of the seed mylk bag is to strain the fiber from liquids, which is especially useful when making nut and seed mylks. These straining bags are also great for making green juice in the blender. You can purchase bags online from raw food support sites, but the easiest thing to do is walk into your local hardware or paint store and ask for a one-gallon paint strainer bag. What you should end up with is a reasonably priced ($2–$6) mesh bag that's perfect for all your liquid straining needs.

DEFINITION

Mylk (instead of "milk") denotes a creamy, fat-based liquid made from raw vegetarian sources such as nuts and seeds.

Heavy-Duty Equipment

Blenders are found in most households and are useful for crushing ice and making simple blended drinks. The raw food detox program employs a number of blended drinks that are delicious and satisfying meals in a glass. Blenders are also useful in this program for making dressings, soups, and sauces. You can choose between a standard, consumer-type blender or one that is more professional. For those willing to make the investment, make a quantum leap in the texture, consistency, and variety of recipes possible by purchasing a high-powered professional blender.

A good, high-powered blender can be costly compared to cheaper consumer blenders, but you may find it to be a worthwhile investment. While $150 is the top-end price for the average consumer blender, a 3-horsepower professional blender can cost from $300 to $500. That seems like a lot of money for something that sits on your countertop and makes drinks. But, by taking the high-powered blender plunge, you can create recipes that could destroy the average consumer blender. The high-powered blender can also blend to a super-smooth consistency and access nutrients by pulverizing plant fiber. The nutritional benefit alone provided by a high-powered blender would pay for itself in health improvement if used to make healthy smoothies and soups on a weekly basis. If you get a chance to test-drive a super blender, experience the difference for yourself.

A food processor might already be hiding in your kitchen cabinet. The advantage of a food processor over a blender is that it works better with dry and moist ingredients. Pesto-type spreads and pâtés are best made in a food processor. If you are preparing food just for yourself, a small-volume food processor will do the trick. When you're feeding more people, a large-volume unit may be better. Most food processors come with three basic blade types: the "S" blade, the slicer blade, and the shredder blade. The "S" blade is used for homogenizing dry and moist ingredients while the other two cut up vegetables and fruits. The shredder and slicer blades are lifesavers when it comes to shredding vegetables such as cabbage and carrots.

Juicers come in a variety of shapes and sizes and are not required for the raw food detox program, but they're very useful. A juicer is special because it separates the fiber from the juice and enables you to experience a nutritious and hydrating drink that's easy to digest.

Citrus juicers work well but are limited to juicing only one type of fruit. When used in conjunction with your blender, you can make citrus smoothies and drinks that will aid you in your detox program.

The spinning basket juicers (centrifuge) are easy to find and are more functional than the citrus juicer. Spinning juicers do well with firm fruits and vegetables. Celery, apples, and carrots fly through a spinning juicer to make an amazing juice.

The next class of juicer is called a masticating juicer because it chews up the item being juiced and forces it through a funneled opening that separates the juice from the fiber. Masticating juicers tend to be more expensive and are typically found at health-food stores or online. Masticating juicers have the added benefit of making nut butters, dough, and frozen desserts (by simply feeding frozen fruit such as bananas or pineapple through the juicer, which comes out on the other end as a smooth sorbet).

Clearing the Decks

To perform this detox program correctly, stock your refrigerator and pantry with delicious raw foods. In many cases, a kitchen is packed full of packaged foods and products that are taking up much-needed space. In the cupboard, the scene is even more interesting—considering that many dry goods have shelf lives just short of eternity. Whether it requires purging the fridge and boxing up what's in the cupboards, make some space. Apply the "out of sight, out of mind" tenet to anything that may tempt you. Replace processed snacks with raw food energy bars and trail mixes. A bowl of fresh fruit should welcome you into your kitchen every morning.

This strategy will go a long way—especially if done prior to beginning the detox program. It's not necessary to do a massive one-day cleaning, although it may be the most effective method. Goal setting is at the heart of this program, so set a date for starting your detox. Give yourself a week or two, depending on how much food is packed into your kitchen. Make an effort to use or give away the tempting foods before your start date arrives. From the moment you set your start date, start filling your fridge and cupboards with raw food detox items.

Stocking Up on Raw Food

The most dramatic change in your food shopping while you are doing the raw food detox involves fresh produce. As simple as it sounds, it's important that fresh produce is actually fresh. This poses a challenge initially, because your visits to the market may need to increase to keep a good supply of the fresh stuff. There are benefits to buying in bulk when it comes to raw food ingredients, but also be careful when buying fresh items in bulk (because you'll need to finish or freeze what you have before it goes bad). With a little experience, your shopping skills will quickly improve.

Fresh Produce

Obviously, fresh produce is at the heart of raw food detox. If you are lucky enough to have a local farmer's market in your area, take advantage of the variety of foods there and the potential for savings. If not, try to buy organic or chemical-free foods when available to avoid toxic residue, and don't be afraid to get to know your vegetables and fruits by touching, squeezing, and smelling before you buy.

For this program, we'll keep your shopping list simple—but for those who are more adventurous or familiar with fresh produce, feel free to add and substitute food items where you see fit. Be sure to check the recipes you'll be making in Part 3 for specific ingredients you might need to buy.

Fruits:

Apples

Bananas

Cherries

Grapefruit

Grapes

Lemons

Limes

Melons

Nectarines

Oranges

Peaches

Pears

Pineapple

Plums

Young Thai coconut

Vegetables:

Avocadoes

Bell peppers—green, red, yellow, and orange

Broccoli

Carrots

Celery

Cauliflower

Collard greens

Cucumber

Garlic

Ginger

Hard squash—spaghetti, butternut, and acorn

Herbs—parsley, cilantro, basil, and so on

Kale

Lettuce (all types)

Onion

Spinach

Tomato

Yellow squash

Zucchini

Refrigerated Items:

Kimchi

Kombucha

Miso

Sauerkraut

Frozen Items:

Coconut, hemp, almond, or cashew "mylk" ice cream

Organic frozen berries and fruits

Organic frozen vegetables—peas, green beans, and corn

Sprouted grain breads

RAWESOME TIP

Coconut, hemp, almond, and cashew "mylk"–based ice creams are now available in many stores. Coconut Bliss is my favorite brand. It's an organic coconut milk–based ice cream that features a variety of exotic flavors. My favorite part about Coconut Bliss is that the ingredient list is short and simple. Choose non-dairy/non-soy ice creams with the least amount of ingredients listed. Avoid non-dairy ice creams that use cane sugar, soy, canola, palm oil, and natural flavor.

Here are some recommended ice cream brands to keep on hand:

- Coconut Bliss/Coconut Milk—Luna and Larry's
- Tempt/Hemp Milk—Living Harvest
- Purely Decadent/Coconut Milk—Turtle Mountain
- Blue Mountain Cashew Creamery/Cashew Milk—Blue Mountain Organics

Dry Goods

Once you make your initial dry-goods purchase, you won't have to buy many of these items for weeks or maybe even months. Like fresh produce, look for organic, toxin-free versions of everything from nuts to oils to soy sauce.

Dried fruit—raisins, apricots, figs, dates, and goji berries

Dulse

Gluten-free pasta

Hiziki

Kelp noodles

Nama shoyu

Raw apple cider vinegar

Raw chocolate bars

Raw, cold-pressed oils—olive, coconut, and sesame

Raw crackers

Raw nori sheets

Raw nut butters

Raw nuts and seeds

Raw snack bars

Quinoa

Superfood powders—spirulina, AFA blue-green algae, and maca

Tamari soy sauce

Wild rice

Sweeteners

Life is sweet, especially if you've got your health. During the raw food detox, it's important to use only whole food, healthy sweeteners. If you are diabetic and must monitor blood sugar, the lower glycemic selections would be best as they will have the least effect on glucose levels. You can check the *glycemic index* of any carbohydrate, including sweeteners, at a number of websites.

DEFINITION

The **glycemic index** is a listing, from 0 to 100, which rates the impact that a carbohydrate has on glucose levels. The lower the number the less effect a carb will have.

Sweeteners:

High Glycemic	Medium Glycemic	Low Glycemic
Acceptable		
Agave nectar	Yacon syrup	Stevia—whole leaf, powder, or extract
Palm sugar	Mesquite powder	Lekanto—from Body Ecology
Coconut syrup		Xylitol—preferably from birch trees
Date paste		
Maple syrup—not raw		
Raw honey—not vegan		

continues

continued

Unacceptable–Do Not Use:

Saccharin—Sweet and Low

Aspartame—Nutrasweet

Sucralose—Splenda

Synthesized stevia—Truvia

White sugar

Raw sugar

Brown sugar

Corn syrup

Beet sugar

Cooked honey—any honey that doesn't say "raw" or "unheated" is most likely cooked

RAWESOME TIP

Dates are an amazing food that can also be used as a sweetener. They are dried fruit that is harvested from a type of palm tree (*Phoenix dactylifera*), and are a calorically dense, fiber- rich food known for benefiting muscle growth, the intestines, heart, sexual function, weight gain, and abdominal cancer.

Date paste can be made by pitting dates and soaking them in water for at least 3 hours. The soaked dates can then be drained and blended into date paste. Some dates farmers use toxic chemicals in their farming practice, so eat only pesticide-free or organic dates when possible. Also, avoid dates that have been chemically preserved.

Easy Mylks

Last but not least, these days it's common to see all types of dairy-free mylks in the dairy section—from almond to coconut to soy. If they're unsweetened and organic, you can certainly enjoy these during your detox. However, making simple dairy-free mylks can be a fun way to use your new equipment and ingredients. Here are three easy recipes to get you started. Simply add all the ingredients to a blender and purée until smooth. You can then flavor your mylks with a healthful sweetener, such as agave or stevia, and add a superfood powder of your choice if desired.

Easy Almond Mylk

2 TB. raw almond butter
2 cups water
Pinch of sea salt

1. Place almond butter, water, and sea salt in a blender. Purée until smooth.

Easy Sesame Mylk

2 TB. raw tahini
2 cups water
Pinch of sea salt

1. Place tahini, water, and sea salt in a blender. Purée until smooth.

Easy Hemp Mylk

¼ cup hemp seeds
2 cups water
Pinch of sea salt

1. Place hemp seeds, water, and sea salt in a blender. Purée until smooth.

The Least You Need to Know

- Knives and a solid cutting board are good basics to have, while other gadgets and light-duty equipment such as peelers, zesters, and slicers can cut down on prep time dramatically.
- Although a high-powered blender can perform many more tasks, a regular commercial blender is fine for the detox program recipes.
- There are a number of different types of juicers you can purchase depending on your budget and long-term goals.
- Making your own "mylks" can be simple and fun.

Raw Food Detox and Social Challenges

In This Chapter

- Getting support from family and friends
- Coping with dining out and going to parties
- Sharing your raw food passion with a partner

Embarking on any special diet plan can pose numerous problems when it comes to socializing with family and friends, but they certainly are not insurmountable. Sometimes, relationships can pose the biggest challenge to a raw food detox success. Staying committed to your program despite temptations and occasional criticism and comments could daunt any detoxer, but this chapter shares advice and suggestions for avoiding these potential pitfalls. Who knows? As you move forward, you may even pick up a few converts along the way!

Family Matters

Announcing you are engaging in a raw food detox is not like coming home with a tattoo, although in some families you may get a similar or even more dramatic response. Because food is at the heart of many family traditions and the choice you've made to do a detox diet may be perceived as disrespectful or threatening to family tradition, there may be a few raised eyebrows. For this reason, some give up before they even begin.

Timing is important. Although modifying your diet before the holiday feast season may be a good idea, the raw food detox program might not. This is especially true if your family is known for being food pushers (for example, "Try some of this" and

"You can't go home without one more piece of such and such"). Try to make your detox as stress-free as possible by taking into consideration any of these types of obstacles you might face and selecting a workable time that will be most conducive to your success.

In many instances, your family will be supportive and even invite you to prepare some of your recipes for them. Consider this a perfect opportunity to share with them what you've learned. Be aware, though, that whatever you prepare may be highly scrutinized. Don't take it personally when relatives pass on your raw food offerings. Some people just aren't ready to experience raw foods beyond salad and a bowl of fruit. Be a shining example of how a healthy detox diet can transform your body and mind for the better.

Social Engagements

Believe it or not, I survived an authentic Italian wedding, in Italy, eating only raw foods. It was quite a challenge, and I don't regret not trying all the amazing food. I did make some exceptions and enjoyed some foods and beverages I normally would have chosen not to eat. Food combining was my first consideration, and quantity was my second consideration.

For the most part, when social gatherings occur, no one really minds if you pass on the wine or even the Brussels sprouts, but if you turn down Aunt Edna's meatloaf, you may be in for big trouble. Be prepared for these challenges. Preparation means knowing what you are going to say and do and sticking with it. Here are some responses to keep in mind to help keep you on the raw food detox path:

- "I'm sorry, I have food allergies and cannot eat that."

- "I'm sorry, I'm gluten and lactose intolerant."

- "I'm on a very strict diet at the moment. I can't eat that, but I'd love to have …"

It's hard to argue with any of these excuses. Always begin by apologizing. If they continue to insist you try a little bit, tell them you could become "very ill." If it is possible to talk to the host ahead of time, you can inform them of your "condition" and ask whether you could bring something of your own. In many cases, they will offer to make something to your liking.

If you are concerned about "making a fuss" and wish to make do with what's available, then be sure to follow these guidelines:

- Food combining first and foremost
- Avoid over indulging on iced drinks, which inhibit digestion and exit times, before meals
- Choose fresh fruits and veggies over breads and pastas
- Stay clear of anything fried
- If there are multiple courses, eat slowly and don't feel obligated to finish everything
- Take enzyme supplements before, during, and after the meal

Another great hint is to arrive satisfied. If you walk into a social gathering that revolves around food and you are hungry, you won't last long. Eat something hearty and healthful before you leave the house, or pack something that will travel well. Pack a superfood smoothie or travel with an avocado and some apples. If you feel your raw food detox program will potentially be derailed by this event, you may want to slide back to an earlier program menu and prepare one of the consciously cooked meals from Program A. A healthful cooked meal may be just what you need to keep your resolve strong.

Finally, have your emergency snacking kit on hand and fully stocked when attending social events. This includes raw salad dressing; healthy, detox-worthy salt; raw snack bars; and travel-friendly fruits and veggies. Even at a traditional barbecue, you should be able to find something you can eat—but don't count on it. If you have invested weeks or months into your raw food detox program, you should be prepared to protect the results of your efforts.

Extended Stays

Part of being a good guest is letting your host be a host. If you're in the midst of the raw food detox program, it may be difficult for you to stay with people for an extended period unless you let them know about your dietary preferences. Do this ahead of time before your host runs out to buy food that he or she thinks you may enjoy. Use your discretion about whether to tell them you have "food allergies" or that you are "on a diet." With food allergies, it is a matter of health, and with a diet, it is a matter of choice. Everyone is familiar with the terms "lactose intolerant" and "gluten allergies." You may get pressured if you tell them what you are doing is a "diet." In the end, it is up to you, but be sure to tell your host in advance. He or she will most likely ask what to pick up for you, so prepare a simple list. You may have the opportunity to do some shopping when you get there as well and perhaps introduce him or her to some delicious raw delicacies.

Raw-Detox Travel

It's possible that you will find yourself traveling at some time during your raw food detox program. Whether it's a short day trip or an extended stay, there are a variety of ways to maintain your diet while traveling. A large number of raw food items travel well. Nuts, seeds, dry fruit, energy bars, trail mix, superfoods, spices, salt, oils, and apple cider vinegar all hold up well on the road or in your luggage. If you're driving, you can load up a cooler with fresh produce and even premade smoothies or juices. You might even consider taking your blender with you when traveling so you can enjoy a daily smoothie breakfast and blended soups in the evening. Traveling like this can save you both time and money.

In the Air

I've been flying raw for years now, and although carry-on restrictions are constantly changing, I've had no problems. On airline flights, you can bring fresh produce on the plane as long as you consume it before you land. This is especially useful on transcontinental and global flights. I usually board the plane with *chlorella tablets*, apples, oranges, celery, and avocados and walk off the plane hydrated and satisfied. Hydration is key while flying, because the pressurized, recycled air in the airplane cabin is effective at dehydrating you and all of the other passengers. Take a pass on all dried and salty snacks while traveling by air and go for fresh fruits, vegetables, and water.

DEFINITION

Chorella tablets are made from single-cell algae, which are naturally whole, nutritious foods that are extremely helpful in removing toxins from the body.

On the Ground

Whether you're flying or driving, once you've arrived at your destination, visit a grocery store to stock up on fresh supplies. Your shopping options will depend on your destination. In major cities, you'll have your pick of grocery stores, health-food stores, and even farmer's markets. Smaller cities will have less variety, but you are likely to find the basics everywhere you go. You can easily look up the shopping options of the place you're going to visit by searching online. Key words such as "organic produce," "health food," and "farmer's market" along with the name of the city should yield some useful results.

> **RAWESOME TIP**
>
> Recently, I traveled to Europe for six weeks and was easily able to maintain my raw food diet with little effort. I was sure to pack superfoods such as goji berries, chlorella, spirulina, maca, and bee pollen along with dates, dry olives, cacao butter, coconut oil, cacao powder, and Himalayan salt. Anything liquid I kept in my checked baggage while the powders and dry foods were fine in my carry-on.

Friends and Colleagues

Raw food detox can give you insight into the caliber of your friends. There was a point in my life when I realized the pointlessness of drinking alcohol. While it took me years of partying and social drinking to come to this conclusion, I was firm in my belief when I arrived at it. Believing in something and actively practicing it are two different things, and that's where the challenge is. Early on during my personal choice to change this aspect of my life, I received both support and pressure from friends. This was all part of the growth for me to see how committed and disciplined I was. Eventually, the pressure no longer affected me, and I was solid in my belief and practice. While the raw food detox program isn't a full-on lifestyle change, it is drastic enough to attract some attention from your friends and colleagues. And while I took months and years to swing back and forth in my commitment and practice, *you* want to do things as quickly and efficiently as possible. To see the best results in the shortest amount of time, stick with the plan as best you can. Be impervious to pressure you may receive from family, friends, and colleagues. Each person's situation is unique, and you'll have to develop a personal plan of action—often in the moment. As long as you are clear about your health goals, firm in your beliefs, and have plenty of delicious raw food staples, you should do fine.

Dining Out

In many ways, the challenges of sticking to your raw food detox program while eating out are similar to those faced when traveling and attending events. Follow those tips, and when you are unsure of what to order, select a salad or salad bar option and you will be on your way toward protecting your detox progress. And if you must, simply eat well before you go out and enjoy the get-together as a social event more than an eating event.

Entertaining Raw

One of the best ways to solicit support for your raw food adventure is to share the new tastes and sensations with others. Why not host a raw food party and open the palates of your friends and family to the fresh and lively flavors of raw food smoothies, entrées, snacks, and desserts?

If "cooking" raw for a crowd is a little too daunting, try combining some of your favorite raw dishes with prepared and purchased dishes so there will be something for everyone. The more people are exposed to the delicious and beneficial detox program you are doing, the more likely they will become staunch allies and perhaps even join you in your endeavor.

Raw Food and Romance

Whether you are single, dating, or hitched, the raw food detox program can have an effect on your interactions with an intimate or potential partner. Because food is often a big part of a couple's co-existence, when one partner is dieting and the other is not, there is more of a chance for friction, frustration, and even ultimate defeat on the dieter's part. Here are some tips to help you maneuver through the intimate implications of your raw food detoxification.

Spousal Support

If you're in an established relationship, you will need the support and understanding of your partner. In most cases, he or she will be very supportive—especially if you don't expect your partner to do the detox diet, too. In some cases, he or she may even join you.

You and your partner should look at the raw food detox program as a win-win situation. You are most likely going to transform your body and your health, which will make you happy (and in turn will make your partner happy). Lay a foundation of support by sharing what you're doing with your spouse and describing the expected results.

Sharing Your Passion

Health and wellness is a great thing to be passionate about. One way to win over (or at least get some respect and support from) friends, family, and spouse is to show them how passionate and committed to personal health you are. Read as much as you can on the subject, and put what interests you into practice. Many people will be curious about what you are doing and how you are feeling. You'll have plenty of opportunities to share your passion for the detox program with everyone.

Raw-Detox Dating

It's not uncommon for a woman to order only a salad for her meal—and it's only a little odd if she packs her own salad dressing. Girls have it easy when it comes to maintaining their rawness; they even have purses in which they can squirrel away all their supplies. Guys, on the other hand, are often expected to eat ridiculously sized portions of meat and starch, and some even consider it "girly" to eat a salad.

So, what do you do if you have a date while you're doing your raw food detox? Stick with the program as much as you can. Most "date-worthy" restaurants have fresh greens on the menu in the form of salads or steamed veggies. If you're a guy doing the raw food detox program, I imagine your date will be more than happy to eat at a restaurant that has fresh options—and if you're a woman, let your date know what your detox diet allows. Think of it as an opportunity to see how patient and supportive your date can be.

Relationships are about shared interests, support, and understanding. If you are having difficulty with any of these, then raw food detox may be the least of your worries. The raw food detox program will be both life-changing and challenging. If you don't have the support and understanding of your partner, you may be in for a difficult and challenging experience. Raw food detox not only cleanses the body physically but also emotionally. This is when you'll need support—or at least, understanding—the most. An easy way to find out whether you have your partner's support is to let him or her know what you're doing, what you hope to achieve, how long you plan on doing the detox diet, and what he or she should expect. Let the person read this book if he or she is willing for clear understanding.

Finding Raw Support

There is an entire community of raw foodists in cities around the world. While your intention may just be to do a month-long raw-detox program, there is still much you can learn and experience by connecting with others who have done "the raw thing." There are a number of online communities that can connect you with raw food folks in your area.

Meetup.com is a worldwide community of groups that have connected because of common interests. Whether you're into ballroom dancing, beekeeping, or bocce ball, you'll be able to find groups of people around the world by entering your zip code or city and your interests. The site is free to join. On Meetup.com, there are hundreds of raw food and healthy-living groups listed around the world. In some major U.S. cities such as New York, Chicago, and Los Angeles, there are multiple raw foods meet-up groups. The groups typically have monthly or even weekly events, such as potlucks, classes, dinners, or movie screenings. The opportunities are limitless in connecting with like-minded people and learning new information about the power of raw foods.

LiveFoodExperience.com is a website I created to provide information and support for those interested in living raw and foods, detox, and sustainable living. The website features my personal blog, recipes, videos, and support items for sale in the online shop.

EightyPercentRaw.com was founded with the intent of bringing together both healthy raw- and cooked-food enthusiasts in one place. The concept is that a person can be extremely healthy and happy consuming 80 percent raw foods and 20 percent cooked foods. EightyPercentRaw.com shares articles, advice, and recipes from several chefs and specialists in the world of health food and healthy living. This free site also has a community forum where members can interact, post experiences, and ask questions.

WeLikeItRaw.com and the online community site GiveItToMeRaw.com (GI2MR) are both free sites loaded with raw food information and support. GI2MR has a very active bulletin board where members engage in discussions on a wide range of topics.

See Appendix D for more on the raw online community and sources for information.

The Least You Need to Know

- Embarking on a detox program can pose challenges to family life and relationships, but with some planning, any challenge can be met.

- Dining out and attending social functions may require bringing specific foods with you and incorporating other strategies to maintain your program.

- Spousal support, although not necessary, can be helpful in sticking to your raw food detox regimen, so share your passion with your partner.

- There are numerous support groups on the Internet and/or in your area that can help you learn more about your detox and enable you to share questions and answers with other like-minded raw food enthusiasts.

Recipes for Success

From lightly cooked beginner's recipes to terrific smoothies and snacks, here you'll find all the recipes you need to perform the raw food detox. No matter which level you decide to begin with, the recipes in this part will serve you well and help you on your quest for vitality and super health. Soups, salads, entrées, and even desserts await you, so tie on your apron and get into the kitchen.

Consciously Cooked Recipes

In This Chapter

- Mouthwatering cooked selections
- Variety vegetables galore
- Easy entrée preparations

Cooked food provides a certain level of comfort and familiarity to many people. I myself still enjoy the comfort provided by eating baked squash on a cold winter night. When cooking is the only option, then choose steamed, boiled, or baked. Stir fry is also acceptable if done lightly and with a high-temperature oil, such as coconut oil, which won't smoke.

When eating a cooked entrée, remember to always start the meal with something fresh and raw, such as a salad with a healthful raw dressing. Also, consider topping a cooked vegetable such as squash with a raw sauce. That will help balance things out (cooked vs. raw), especially early in your detox program. Also, try topping cooked pasta with the raw marinara sauce or marinated vegetables and mushrooms for a terrific meal. Get creative and enjoy your meals, even the cooked ones, with raw gusto!

Baked Spaghetti Squash

Mildly flavored and fun to eat, spaghetti squash is baked to fork tender and topped with delicious, tangy orange and miso–marinated vegetables and sauce.

Yield:	Serving size:	Prep time:	Cook time:
2 halves	1 squash half	10 minutes	50 minutes

1 medium spaghetti squash
½ cup water
2 servings (about 4 cups) Marinated Veggies (recipe in Chapter 12)
2 servings (about 2 TB.) Almond Miso Sauce (recipe in Chapter 10)

1. Preheat the oven to 375°F. Cut squash in half lengthwise and scoop out seeds. Place squash halves cut-side down on a rimmed baking sheet and pour water around the edges.

2. Bake until inside of squash is fork tender, about 45 minutes. Use a fork to carefully scrape the "spaghetti" up from the skin and transfer to a mixing bowl. Set squash shell aside for serving. Turn off the oven.

3. Toss Marinated Veggies with squash, then transfer mixture into reserved squash shells evenly, and return to the warm oven for 5 minutes.

4. When ready to serve, drizzle with Almond Miso Sauce.

Baked Acorn Squash

Everyone's favorite winter squash gets a tasty filling of veggies and a lively and nutty cheese-flavored sauce.

Yield:	Serving size:	Prep time:	Cook time:
2 halves	1 squash half	10 minutes	35 minutes

1 large acorn squash

½ cup water

2 servings (about 4 cups)Marinated Veggies (recipe in Chapter 12)

2 servings (about ½ cup) Cheezy Sauce (recipe in Chapter 10)

1. Preheat the oven to 375°F. Cut squash in half lengthwise and scoop out seeds. Place halves cut-side down on a rimmed baking sheet and pour water around the edges.

2. Bake until inside of squash is fork tender, about 30 minutes. Turn off the oven.

3. Flip over squash halves and fill each with Marinated Veggies. Return to the warm oven for 5 minutes.

4. When ready to serve, drizzle with Cheezy Sauce.

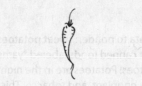

RAWESOME TIP

Taking digestive enzyme tablets before each meal—cooked or raw—will optimize your digestion. This is especially important when eating cooked food on program A. Look for enzyme tablets at your health-food store and follow the dosage on the box.

Baked Sweet Potato

Simple, delicious, and satisfying, baked sweet potatoes are a great transition food for beginning and ending a detox program.

Yield:	Serving size:	Prep time:	Cook time:
1 sweet potato	1 sweet potato	5 minutes	40–60 minutes

1 large sweet potato
1 TB. coconut oil
1 garlic clove, minced
Pinch of sea salt

1. Preheat the oven to 400°F.
2. Poke sweet potato multiple times with a fork to aerate. Place sweet potato directly on the oven rack and bake until fork tender, about 40 to 60 minutes.
3. Remove sweet potato from oven and allow to cool to room temperature. Cut in half, drizzle with coconut oil, and top with garlic and sea salt.

Variation: You can boil sweet potatoes and then mash them as well. Use coconut oil, salt, palm sugar, cloves, and cinnamon to make it a festive treat.

FRESH FACT

Here's some raw data to ponder: sweet potatoes aren't even related to white potatoes, and most canned foods labeled "yams" technically aren't yams—they're sweet potatoes! Potatoes are in the nightshade family along with tomatoes, peppers, eggplant, and tobacco. This family of plant contains toxic compounds known as glykoalkaloids, concentrated in the leaves, fruits, and roots. Cooking helps neutralize these toxins in white potatoes to safe levels. Sweet potatoes, however, being unrelated, are safe to eat both raw and cooked.

Comparison of Baked Sweet Potato, Russet Potato, and Red Potato (with skin on) from NutritionData.com

	Sweet Potato	Russet Potato	Red Potato
Weight	200 grams	299 grams	299 grams
Protein	4g, at 299g = 6g	8g	7g
Vitamin A	769% RDA	1% RDA	1% RDA
Vitamin C	65% RDA	64% RDA	63% RDA
Iron	8% RDA	18% RDA	12% RDA
Calcium	8% RDA	5% RDA	3% RDA
Glycemic Index (GI)	17	29	26
Inflammatory #	378	–177	–157
Nutrient Balance	65	51	51
Protein Quality	82	75	92

The lower the "GI" number, the better. Positive "Inflammatory" numbers mean the food is considered an anti-inflammatory. The higher the "Nutrient Balance" and "Protein Quality," the better.

Steamed Veggies

This cooking method will be a favorite for all your cooked veggies, especially when topped with the accompanying tangy sauce.

Yield:	Serving size:	Prep time:	Cook time:
About 4 cups	About 2 cups	20 minutes	12 minutes

2 small red or white potatoes

2 medium zucchini, ends trimmed

1 small onion, peeled and trimmed

1 red or orange bell pepper, halved and seeded

2 servings (about ½ cup) 5 Easy Pieces sauce (recipe in Chapter 10)

1. Chop potatoes, zucchini, onion, and pepper into small, bite-size pieces, keeping the potatoes separate.

2. Using a stainless-steel vegetable steamer or sieve set over a pot of simmering water, steam potatoes first, covered, for about 4 minutes. Add zucchini, peppers, and onion and steam, covered, for another 5 to 8 minutes until all vegetables are nearly fork tender.

3. Remove from heat and allow to cool. Top with 5 Easy Pieces sauce.

Variation: Enjoy the steamed veggies and sauce wrapped in raw nori (seaweed) sheets or crisp cabbage or romaine leaves.

RAWESOME TIP

Save the water used for vegetable steaming in the refrigerator for up to two days and use it in soups or other recipes to get every last nutrient.

Portobello Bella Bella

Hearty and satisfying portobello mushroom caps are flavored with savory tamari soy sauce and a bit of lemon and parsley.

Yield:	Serving size:	Prep time:	Cook time:
2 mushroom caps	1 mushroom cap	15 minutes	10 minutes

2 large portobello tops, gills scraped away with a spoon and discarded

1 small sweet onion, diced

1 red bell pepper, seeded and diced

2 TB. olive oil

1 TB. soy sauce

2 tsp. lemon juice or apple cider vinegar

2 TB. fresh parsley, minced

1. Preheat the oven to 350°F. Place mushroom caps cavity-side up on a baking sheet.

2. In a medium mixing bowl, combine onion, bell pepper, olive oil, soy sauce, and lemon juice or apple cider vinegar and spoon half the mixture into each mushroom cap. Bake in the oven for 10 minutes.

3. Cool to room temperature and serve topped with minced parsley.

Variation: For those of you who have a dehydrator, make this recipe raw by dehydrating the stuffed mushroom for 2 hours at 115°F to 120°F.

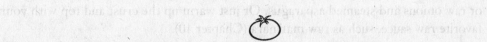

Veggie Pizza

Amazing but true, pizza is back on the menu with this lightly cooked rendition that features a colorful and tasty variety of super-healthful vegetables.

Yield:	Serving size:	Prep time:	Cook time:
1 pizza	½ a pizza	20 minutes	12 minutes

1 gluten-free, organic 10- or 12-inch prebaked pizza crust

1 small red bell pepper, cored and diced

1 small yellow bell pepper, cored and diced

2 cups fresh spinach leaves, roughly chopped

1 cup raw green olives, pitted and chopped

2 TB. olive oil

1 tsp. sea salt

2 large ripe tomatoes, sliced

¼ cup fresh basil leaves, minced

1. Follow the package directions for pizza crust and preheat the oven.

2. Combine red pepper, yellow pepper, spinach, olives, olive oil, and sea salt in a medium bowl and toss well to combine. Evenly distribute vegetable mixture over pizza crust and bake according to directions.

3. Remove from oven and let cool before topping with tomatoes and basil. Serve immediately.

Variation: Try topping your pizza with marinated mushrooms or veggies (Chapter 12) or raw onions and steamed asparagus. Or just warm up the crust and top with your favorite raw sauce, such as raw marinara (Chapter 10).

Pasta Party

When cooked pasta is your craving, this easy and quick Asian-inspired dish with the creaminess of almond butter and the tang of ginger will definitely satisfy.

Yield:	Serving size:	Prep time:	Cook time:
About 4 cups	About 2 cups	10 minutes	10 minutes

½ lb. gluten-free pasta, brown rice, or *quinoa*

1½ TB. miso

2 TB. almond butter

1 TB. tamari soy sauce

1 garlic clove, minced

¼ tsp. minced fresh ginger

¼ cup chopped scallions (about 2)

1. Cook pasta or grain according to the package directions, drain, and set aside in a bowl to cool to room temperature.

2. In a small mixing bowl, whisk together miso, almond butter, tamari soy sauce, garlic, and ginger.

3. Pour sauce over pasta and toss gently to coat. Sprinkle with scallions and serve.

Variation: Turn this dish totally raw by using a spiral slicer to make zucchini threads or use purchased kelp noodles.

 DEFINITION

Quinoa is a Peruvian grain that is gluten-free and is an excellent source of protein. You can find it in the rice section of your grocery store.

Wild Rice Medley

Nutty and delicious wild rice stars in this dish, which is enhanced with a sweet dressing, aromatic vegetables, and mushrooms.

Yield:	Serving size:	Prep time:	Cook time:
About 4 cups	About 1 cup	15 minutes	40 minutes

3 cups water

¼ tsp. sea salt

1 cup wild rice

1 (6 oz.) package dried mushrooms

1 TB. lemon juice

1 TB. miso

1 tsp. olive or sesame oil

1 tsp. palm sugar or agave nectar

1 tsp. tamari soy sauce

2 garlic cloves, minced

¼ cup shredded carrots

¼ cup finely diced celery

1. Bring water to a boil over high heat. Stir in salt and wild rice, cover, reduce the heat to low, and cook until tender, about 40 minutes.

2. Meanwhile, soak dried mushrooms in a bowl with a little water. In another bowl, whisk together lemon juice, miso, olive or sesame oil, palm sugar or agave, and tamari soy sauce and stir into mushrooms. Set aside.

3. When rice is cooked, remove from heat and cool for 5 minutes. Stir in mushroom mixture along with garlic, carrots, and celery and allow to come to room temperature before serving.

Variation: Spice up your rice with a little cayenne pepper, paprika, or chili powder. Or add other vegetables such as diced zucchini, tomatoes, and peppers. Firmer vegetables such as cauliflower and broccoli can be directly added to the pot of rice after it has come off the heat.

FRESH FACT

Wild rice is actually not a rice at all but a type of grass. Its nutritional impact and fiber value is greater than both white and brown rices.

Sprouted Bread Toast Toppers

Although these toppings require no cooking, whole-grain bread, even if it contains sprouts, counts as a "cooked" selection. Enjoy each of the following suggestions any time of day, or simply spread a little organic butter on your toast for a satisfying treat when you are hankering for the taste of bread.

Morning Slice

Yield:	Serving size:	Prep time:
2 slices	2 bread slices with toppings	5 minutes

2 slices sprouted bread, toasted if desired

2 TB. almond butter

2 tsp. miso

1½ tsp. water

1 banana, peeled and sliced

1 tsp. cinnamon

1. In a small bowl, mix together almond butter, miso, and water to make a paste. Spread onto slices of bread.

2. Top bread slices with banana and sprinkle with cinnamon.

Midday Slice

Yield:	Serving size:	Prep time:
2 slices	2 bread slices with toppings	5 minutes

2 slices sprouted bread, toasted if desired

1 avocado, halved, seeded, and scooped from outer skin

1 TB. miso

½ medium tomato, sliced

¼ medium onion, sliced

2 lettuce leaves, shredded

1. In a small bowl, mix together avocado and miso to form a paste. Spread onto bread slices.

2. Top with tomato, onion, and lettuce to make 2 open-faced sandwiches or put together for 1 hearty sandwich.

Evening Slice

Yield:	Serving size:	Prep time:
2 slices	2 bread slices with toppings	5 minutes

2 slices sprouted bread, toasted if desired

2 TB. Cashew Cheeze (recipe in Chapter 10)

1 marinated portobello mushroom cap (from the Stuffed Portobello recipe in Chapter 12)

½ medium tomato, sliced

¼ medium onion, sliced

2 lettuce leaves, shredded

1. Spread 1 tablespoon Cashew Cheeze on each bread slice.

2. Place mushroom cap, whole or sliced, on 1 slice bread and top with tomato, onion, and lettuce.

3. Top with remaining bread slice, gently press down, cut in half, and serve immediately.

DETOXER'S ALERT

If at any point in your detox diet you feel the effects of a strong cleansing reaction, then try drinking a glass of purified water, consider colon hydrotherapy, or eat one of the cooked food recipes in this chapter. The baked sweet potato is always a good choice.

Raw Spreads, Sauces, and Dressings

In This Chapter

- Delicious and nutritious spreads
- Saucing up your veggies
- In the raw and dressed up too

The recipes in this chapter will become some of your favorite kitchen creations once you taste the terrific results. From simple spreads for crackers and bread to dynamic dressings for every type of salad, you'll enjoy every bite as you embark on your raw detox journey.

5 Easy Pieces

This terrific hemp and miso combination (plus three other ingredients) is the basis for a great spread or sauce that can be thinned or embellished depending on your preference.

Yield:	Serving size:	Prep time:
1 cup	¼ cup or more	10 minutes

¾ cup hemp seeds

3 TB. apple cider vinegar

3 TB. miso

⅓ cup olive oil

Sea salt to taste

¼ to ¾ cups water

1. Combine hemp seed, apple cider vinegar, miso, olive oil, and sea salt in a blender and purée until smooth. Add as little or as much water as needed for desired thickness.

Variation: Substitute tahini or almond butter for the hemp seeds, orange juice for the vinegar, or use a flavored type of miso. You can also add fresh herbs, garlic, or any number of spices—but you'll need to rename your sauce!

Almond Miso Spread/Sauce

Easy and quick to make, this simple spread is great on apple slices or celery and also as a tasty sauce for raw or steamed veggies.

Yield:	Serving size:	Prep time:
4 TB.	1 heaping TB. or more	8 minutes

¼ cup almond butter

2 TB. miso

1 to 2 tsp. lemon juice

1 tsp. to ¼ cup water

1. Combine almond butter, miso, and lemon juice in a bowl and mix with a spoon to a creamy paste. Add water as desired to thin the consistency.

Sesame Spread/Sauce

Delicious sesame-flavored tahini is featured in this great spread (or sauce) with a hint of pungent garlic.

Yield:	Serving size:	Prep time:
4 TB.	1 heaping TB. or more	10 minutes

¼ cup tahini

1 TB. miso

1 TB. lemon juice or apple cider vinegar

1 tsp. tamari soy sauce

1 garlic clove, minced

2 TB. to ¼ cup water

1. Combine tahini, miso, lemon juice or apple cider vinegar, tamari soy sauce, and garlic in a blender and purée until smooth. Thin with water as desired.

Variation: "Heat" it up with the addition of a little curry powder and/or cayenne pepper.

Cheezy Sauce

Choose cashews or hemp seeds as the base for this fabulous sauce (that can also be used as a spread) that gets its "cheezy" flavor from nutritional yeast.

Yield:	Serving size:	Prep time:
1 cup	About ¼ cup or more	15 minutes

½ cup cashews or hemp seeds

1 medium red or orange bell pepper, seeded and diced

2 TB. nutritional yeast

1 TB. miso

1 to 2 tsp. lemon juice or apple cider vinegar

Sea salt to taste

2 TB. to ¼ cup water

1. Combine cashews or hemp seeds, bell pepper, yeast, miso, lemon juice or apple cider vinegar, and sea salt in a blender or food processor and purée until smooth. Thin with water to desired consistency.

FRESH FACT

Nutritional yeast is a type of deactivated yeast that is popular with vegetarians and vegans because of its cheeselike flavor and healthful content.

Classic Marinara

This tomato-based sauce, which is ideal over pasta in program A, is also terrific over veggie or kelp noodles as well as your choice of fresh steamed or raw vegetables.

Yield:	Serving size:	Prep time:
About 1⅓ cups	About ⅓ cup	25 minutes

1 cup sun-dried tomatoes, soaked, drained, and chopped
½ cup diced fresh tomatoes
1 TB. olive oil
1 TB. apple cider vinegar or lemon juice
1 TB. minced fresh Italian herbs, such as basil and oregano
½ tsp. sea salt or to taste

1. Combine sun-dried tomatoes, fresh tomatoes, olive oil, apple cider vinegar or lemon juice, Italian herbs, and sea salt in a medium bowl and stir until well mixed. Serve immediately.

Variations:

Dulse Marinara: Stir in 2 tablespoons dulse flakes.

Creamy Marinara: Add ½ cup soaked cashews or hemp seeds and 2 tablespoons nutritional yeast and combine in the blender or food processor.

FRESH FACT

Dulse, which is similar to seaweed, has a very high protein content and even contains all trace minerals required by the human body. Look for it in your health-food store.

Pumpkin Seed Pesto

Fresh aromatic basil and raw green pumpkin seeds combine for this thick pesto sauce that's great with salads and all veggies, cooked or raw.

Yield:	Serving size:	Prep time:
About 1½ cups	About ¼ cup	25 minutes

1 cup green pumpkin seeds

¼ cup olive oil

¼ cup fresh basil leaves, firmly packed

2 TB. diced onion

2 tsp. lemon juice

½ tsp. sea salt or to taste

1 TB. miso (optional)

1. Combine pumpkin seeds, olive oil, basil, onion, lemon juice, sea salt, and miso (if using) in a blender or food processor and purée until smooth. Transfer to a sealable container and refrigerate or use immediately.

Cashew Cheeze

If you're really missing the flavor of cheese, whip up this great alternative and serve with raw veggies and fruit.

Yield:	Serving size:	Prep time:
About 12 TB.	About 2 TB.	10 minutes

1 cup cashews, soaked in water for 30 minutes

¼ cup olive oil

1 TB. miso

1 TB. nutritional yeast, or more to taste

2 tsp. apple cider vinegar or lemon juice

Sea salt to taste

1. Drain cashews and add along with olive oil, miso, yeast, apple cider vinegar or lemon juice, and sea salt to a food processor and purée until smooth.

2. Add more nutritional yeast to get a thicker, nuttier, and cheesier consistency.

Simple Miso Marinade

Use this as a flavorful base marinade for any veggies (especially mushrooms), and consider making a large batch to marinate a supply of veggies for the week.

Yield:	Serving size:	Prep time:
About ½ cup	2 TB.	15 minutes

3 TB. miso
¼ cup lemon juice
¼ cup olive oil
2 tsp. palm sugar or agave nectar
1 tsp. tamari soy sauce
1 garlic clove, minced

1. Blend or whisk together miso, lemon juice, olive oil, palm sugar or agave, tamari soy sauce, and garlic. Transfer to a sealable container, add your choice of vegetables, and shake vigorously. If marinating for more than 2 hours, refrigerate.

2. Shake container periodically to coat. Keep up to 1 week.

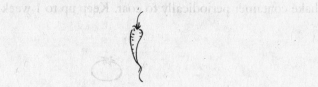

Orange Miso Marinade

Soy-free chickpea miso is the base for this terrific marinade that blends well with the flavors of orange and ginger.

Yield:	Serving size:	Prep time:
About ¾ cup	About ¼ cup	15 minutes

¼ cup chickpea miso

¼ cup olive oil

¼ cup orange juice

2 TB. apple cider vinegar

2 tsp. tamari soy sauce

2 garlic cloves, minced

2 tsp. minced fresh ginger

1. Blend or whisk together chickpea miso, olive oil, orange juice, apple cider vinegar, tamari soy sauce, garlic, and ginger. Transfer to a sealable container, add your choice of vegetables, and shake vigorously. If marinating for more than 2 hours, refrigerate.

2. Shake container periodically to coat. Keep up to 1 week.

BBQ Marinade

Just a few additions turn the Orange Miso Marinade into a great-tasting barbecue that's tangy, sweet, and flavorful.

Yield:	Serving size:	Prep time:
About 1 cup	About ¼ cup	15 minutes

½ cup sun-dried tomatoes, chopped and soaked in water for 20 minutes
1 recipe (about ¾ cup) Orange Miso Marinade (recipe in Chapter 10)
1 TB. palm sugar or 2 pitted dates
2 tsp. paprika or chili powder

1. Drain sun-dried tomatoes and reserve liquid.

2. Place sun-dried tomatoes, Orange Miso Marinade, palm sugar or dates, and paprika or chili powder in a food processor or blender and purée until smooth. If marinade is too thick, add reserved liquid from sun-dried tomatoes.

3. Transfer to a sealable container, add your choice of vegetables, and shake vigorously. If marinating for more than 2 hours, refrigerate.

4. Shake container periodically to coat. Keep up to 1 week.

Garlic Avo Dressing

You'll love this creamy dressing on your tossed green salad with a hint of hot pepper and the pungency of garlic.

Yield:	Serving size:	Prep time:
About 1 cup	About ¼ cup	20 minutes

1 avocado, halved, seeded, scooped from outer skin, and diced

1 TB. miso

½ cup water

½ cup olive oil

½ cup diced onion

¼ cup lemon juice or apple cider vinegar

1 small jalapeno pepper, seeded and diced

2 garlic cloves, minced

Sea salt to taste

1. Combine avocado, miso, water, olive oil, onion, lemon juice or apple cider vinegar, hot pepper, garlic, and sea salt in a blender and purée until smooth. Transfer to a sealable container and keep refrigerated for up to 3 days.

Apricot Vinaigrette

The sweetness of apricots and the unique flavor of tarragon make this delicious dressing perfect for salads and cut-up raw veggies.

Yield:	Serving size:	Prep time:
About 1½ cups	About ¼ cup	20 minutes

1 cup dried apricots, soaked in ¾ cup water for at least 30 minutes

1 cup olive oil

¼ cup apple cider vinegar

1 TB. minced fresh tarragon

½ tsp. sea salt or to taste

1. Combine apricots, olive oil, apple cider vinegar, tarragon, and sea salt in a blender or food processor and purée or pulse until smooth. Transfer to a sealable container and keep refrigerated for up to 1 week.

Variation: Replace apricots with dried figs.

FRESH FACT

Fresh and dried figs are one of the healthiest fruits available. They are one of the highest plant sources of calcium, copper, manganese, magnesium, potassium, vitamin K, and fiber. Figs are rich in antioxidants, flavonoids, and polyphenols. Fresh or dried figs are amazing.

Avocado Dressing

This is a great standard, creamy avocado dressing—reminiscent of guacamole—that you'll be whipping up often.

Yield:	Serving size:	Prep time:
About 1 cup	About ¼ cup	25 minutes

1 avocado, halved, seeded, scooped from outer skin, and chopped

¼ cup diced onion

2 TB. lime juice or apple cider vinegar

2 small celery stalks, trimmed and chopped

2 TB. fresh cilantro leaves

½ tsp. sea salt or to taste

2 TB. nutritional yeast (optional)

1. Combine avocado, onion, lime juice or apple cider vinegar, celery, cilantro, sea salt, and yeast (if using) in a blender and purée until smooth. Transfer to a sealable container and refrigerate for up to 3 days.

Variation: Add half a medium red bell pepper, seeded and diced; a pinch of cayenne pepper; and a minced garlic clove for a kicked-up version.

Spirulina Power Dressing

Super spirulina is the powerful ingredient in this dressing, which is super delicious and will do your detoxing body a lot of good.

Yield:	Serving size:	Prep time:
8–12 TB.	2–3 TB.	10 minutes

½ cup olive oil

¼ cup spirulina

¼ cup dulse

2 TB. apple cider vinegar

1 garlic clove, minced

1 TB. maca

½ tsp. sea salt

1. Whisk or blend together olive oil, spirulina, dulse, apple cider vinegar, garlic, maca, and sea salt and serve immediately or store in a sealable container at room temperature for up to 2 days.

FRESH FACT

Spirulina, or blue-green algae, although a popular health food today, was actually a staple whole food for the Aztecs through the sixteenth century.

Raw Soups and Salads

In This Chapter

- Soups for sustenance and satisfaction
- "Floaters" make the meal
- Sensational and unusual salads

If you've ever enjoyed a bowl of gazpacho, you already know how refreshing and flavorful a raw soup can be. In this chapter, you'll meet some terrific, standard raw soups that can be eaten cold or even lightly warmed depending on your preference. From crispy cucumbers to exotic curry, you'll enjoy a variety of tastes and experiences.

If you've ever topped a bowl of soup with a sprinkling of cheese or crackers, you're already familiar with the idea of "floaters"—a great addition to any soup. In this chapter, you'll get some super ideas for creating interesting and healthy raw floaters for a superb bowl of nourishment.

Although salads may seem an obvious choice for raw food detoxification, the salad recipes you'll find here are a great medley of classics with a twist and some unexpected taste experiences from a variety of ingredients. Enjoy all of them as you detox your way to great health.

Cucumber Dill Soup

Super hydrating and wonderfully delicious, the fresh flavor of cucumber gets creamy with the help of avocado in this classic soup with a lemony twist.

Yield:	Serving size:	Prep time:
3 cups	1 ½ cups	20 minutes

2 cups cucumbers, roughly chopped

1 cup water

¼ cup lemon juice

1 avocado, halved, seeded, scooped from outer skin, and diced

¼ cup fresh dill sprigs (or 1 TB. dried)

¼ cup diced onion

¼ tsp. sea salt or more to taste

1. Combine cucumbers, water, lemon juice, avocado, dill, onion, and sea salt in a blender and purée until smooth. Serve chilled or at room temperature.

Simple Miso Soup

Japanese miso soup can be wonderfully satisfying and comforting while being a real snap to make. Enjoy warm or at room temperature.

Yield:	Serving size:	Prep time:
About 1 cup	About 1 cup	5 minutes

2 TB. miso

1 cup water

¼ cup lemon juice

¼ cup chopped scallions

1. Whisk or blend together miso, water, and lemon juice. Sprinkle with scallions and serve.

RAWESOME TIP

How do you turn a simple soup into a meal? With floaters, of course! Floaters are any fresh goodies that you cut and add to your soup just before serving. Here's a list of ideas to inspire you:

Avocado cubes	Green onions
Bell pepper bits	Hemp seeds
Celery slices	Fresh herbs
Carrot shreds	Kelp noodles
Corn kernels	Mushroom slices
Dulse flakes	Tomato cubes
Flax cracker crumbs	

Almond Miso Soup

Sweet and creamy almond butter adds another flavor element to delicious miso soup topped with some colorful "floaters."

Yield:	Serving size:	Prep time:
About 1 cup	About 1 cup	10 minutes

1 serving (about 1 cup) Simple Miso Soup (recipe in Chapter 11)

2 TB. almond butter

2 tsp. maca

1 garlic clove, minced

Sea salt to taste

½ cup diced bell pepper (any color)

2 TB. chopped fresh parsley leaves

1. Whisk or blend together Simple Miso Soup, almond butter, maca, garlic, and sea salt until smooth. Pour into a serving bowl and top with bell pepper and parsley.

Sea Veggie Soup

The flavor of the sea enhances a simple miso soup with the addition of some flavorful Japanese ingredients.

Yield:	Serving size:	Prep time:
About 1 cup	About 1 cup	10 minutes

1 serving (about 1 cup) Simple Miso Soup (recipe in Chapter 11)

2 TB. dulse flakes

2 TB *hiziki*, soaked in water for 20 minutes

2 TB. arame or kelp, soaked in water for 20 minutes

1 tsp. tamari soy sauce

½ cup diced bell pepper (any color)

1. To the Simple Miso Soup, stir in dulse flakes and soaked and drained hiziki and arame or kelp.

2. Stir in tamari soy sauce and float bell pepper on top just before serving.

Variation: For a creamy version, blend in half an avocado when preparing the Simple Miso Soup.

> **DEFINITION**
>
> **Hiziki** is a brown sea vegetable that grows wild and has been a staple of the Japanese diet for centuries. It contains a good amount of fiber, calcium, iron, iodine, and magnesium.

Sesame Curry Soup

Delicious sesame-flavored tahini and the pizzazz of curry make this miso soup version an exotic winner.

Yield:	Serving size:	Prep time:
About 1 cup	About 1 cup	10 minutes

1 serving, about 1 cup, Simple Miso Soup (recipe in Chapter 11)

2 TB. tahini

2 tsp. curry powder

¼ cup diced onion

Sea salt to taste

1 TB. *each* chopped fresh parsley and cilantro leaves

1. Combine Simple Miso Soup, tahini, curry powder, onion, and sea salt in a blender and purée until smooth. Serve topped with parsley and cilantro.

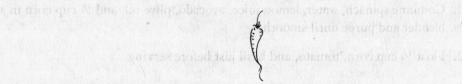

 RAWESOME TIP

When heating soup, be sure not to allow the temperature to go higher than 118°F. Set a probe thermometer in the pot when heating on the stovetop, stir constantly, and remove the soup from the heat source when the temperature reaches 115°F to allow for "carry-over" cooking.

Spinach Soup

A medley of freshness, this soup is a real treat—especially in the summer when tomatoes and corn are at their peak. Get creative and make your own seasonal floaters when inspired by fresh produce.

Yield:	Serving size:	Prep time:
About 2 cups	About 1 cup	20 minutes

2 cups fresh spinach leaves, firmly packed

1 or 1½ cups water to thin

¼ cup lemon juice

1 avocado, halved, seeded, scooped from outer skin, and diced

1 TB. olive oil

½ cup fresh corn kernels, divided

1 medium tomato, diced

¼ cup fresh basil leaves, minced

1. Combine spinach, water, lemon juice, avocado, olive oil, and ¼ cup corn in a blender and purée until smooth.

2. Float ¼ cup corn, tomato, and basil just before serving.

G-Man's Coconut Soup

My friends Gary and Kiki really get the credit for this brilliant and delicious soup that lends itself to myriad variations.

Yield:	Serving size:	Prep time:
About 2 cups	About 1 cup	30 minutes

1 young Thai coconut, meat and water

1 cup water

1 TB. miso

1 TB. tamari soy sauce or Nama Shoyu miso

1 TB. sesame oil

1 TB. toasted sesame oil

1 TB. apple cider vinegar

2 TB. hot pepper–infused olive oil

1 tsp. store-bought "Thai spice blend" or other spice blend

2 garlic cloves, peeled

1 one-inch piece fresh ginger

½ cup diced onion

1 avocado, halved, seeded, scooped from outer skin

1 TB. nutritional yeast

¼ tsp. cayenne pepper

1 cup corn kernels

½ cup diced tomato

½ cup diced bell pepper (any color)

½ cup chopped scallions

1 cup kelp noodles

1. Add coconut, water, miso, tamari soy sauce or Nama Shoyu, sesame oils, apple cider vinegar, hot olive oil, Thai spices, garlic, ginger, onion, avocado, yeast, and cayenne pepper to the blender and purée until smooth.

2. Transfer purée to a bowl and stir in corn, tomato, pepper, scallions, and kelp noodles. Serve cold or warm.

Variation: Try adding other international flavors, such as sun-dried tomatoes, garam masala, curry, and Mexican or Italian seasonings in place of the Thai spice blend.

FRESH FACT

Garam masala is an Indian spice blend that features cinnamon and that is usually added to a curried dish at the end of cooking for aromatic purposes.

Creamy Cauliflower Ses'same Soup

Yield:	Serving size:	Prep time:
2 cups	1 cup	15 minutes

Super easy to make and delicious going down, you'll love this creamy soup any time of day.

Reserved liquid (about 1 cup) from cauliflower cous cous (see Curry Cauliflower Cous Cous recipe later in chapter)

1 cup water

1 avocado, halved, pitted, and removed from peel

2 TB. miso

¼ cup yellow onion

½ cup diced orange pepper

¼ tsp. toasted sesame oil

1 TB. olive oil

1 tsp. chia

1 tsp. of Thai spice blend, or another spice blend

1 TB. green pepper, diced

Dash paprika

1 TB. crumbled raw-friendly crackers

1. Place cauliflower couscous liquid, water, ½ avocado, miso, onion, pepper, oils, chia, and spice blend into blender and blend until combined. Dice remaining avocado and set aside.

2. Garnish with diced avocado, green pepper, paprika, and cracker crumbles.

Massaged Kale

Healthy kale is the base for this easy-to-make salad that can be topped with any number of diced raw veggies.

Yield:	Serving size:	Prep time:
4–6 cups	2–3 cups	15 minutes

2 bunches kale, stemmed, washed, and dried

2 tsp. sea salt

2 large tomatoes, diced

1 avocado, halved, seeded, scooped from outer skin, and diced

Fresh lemon or lime juice, to taste

Olive oil to taste

1. Place kale leaves in a large bowl and sprinkle with salt. Using clean hands, "massage" the leaves by squeezing and tearing kale with salt for 5 minutes. (Kale will become wilted and limp.)

2. Add tomatoes, avocado, lemon or lime juice, and olive oil and toss gently before serving.

RAWESOME TIP

Be sure to save kale stems and other edible vegetable trimmings for juicing. Store in the refrigerator and wash just before using.

Sea Veggie Salad

Here's a terrifically refreshing and flavorful salad—both salty and sweet and perfect at lunch or dinner.

Yield:	Serving size:	Prep time:
About 3 cups	About 1½ cups	20 minutes

¼ cup hiziki, soaked in water for 20 minutes

¼ cup nori leaves, broken up and soaked in water for 20 minutes

1 medium cucumber, trimmed and finely diced

2 medium apples, cored and finely diced

2 medium celery stalks, trimmed and finely diced

2 TB. dulse flakes

1 TB. minced fresh ginger

2 TB. miso

1 TB. olive oil or sesame oil

¼ tsp. cayenne pepper or paprika

Sea salt to taste

1. Drain hiziki and nori and combine with cucumber, apples, celery stalks, dulse flakes, ginger, miso, olive oil or sesame oil, cayenne pepper or paprika, and sea salt in a mixing bowl, combining thoroughly with your hands. Serve immediately.

FRESH FACT

Nori contains high amounts of protein, iodine, carotene, calcium, and iron. Raw nori sheets are black in appearance while toasted nori sheets have a greenish color.

Eggless Egg Salad

Black salt is the secret ingredient in this surprisingly egg salad–tasting dish that's loaded with nutrition and can also be used as a dip or spread.

Yield:	Serving size:	Prep time:
About 1⅓ cups	About ⅔ cup	20 minutes

1 cup sunflower or pumpkin seeds

3 TB. apple cider vinegar

¼ cup water

¼ cup olive oil

1 tsp. turmeric

2 tsp Kala Namak (black salt)

2 medium celery stalks, trimmed and finely diced

½ cup finely diced yellow bell pepper

1 avocado, halved, seeded, scooped from outer skin, and cubed

1 medium tomato, diced

Cabbage or romaine lettuce leaves, for serving

1. Combine sunflower or pumpkin seeds, vinegar, water, oil, turmeric, and Kala Namak in a blender or food processor and purée to a paste.

2. Transfer mixture to a medium bowl and mix in celery, bell pepper, avocado, and tomato, stirring gently.

3. Serve spoonfuls wrapped in cabbage or romaine lettuce leaves if desired.

DEFINITION

Black Indian salt is also known as **Kala Namak.** It typically has a light-pink or purple color, and because of impurities such as sulfur, it smells and tastes like eggs. This special salt is used in Indian cuisine and can be purchased online or at a local Indian market.

Tu-No Salad

The texture and a hint of familiar flavor, not unlike a traditional tuna salad, is the attraction in this terrific dish that can be served as a dip or spread on crackers or in lettuce leaves.

Yield:	Serving size:	Prep time:
About 1⅓ cups	About ⅔ cup	20 minutes

1 cup sunflower or green pumpkin seeds, soaked in water for 1 hour and rinsed

3 TB. lemon juice or apple cider vinegar

1 TB. miso

¼ cup olive oil

1 cup celery stalks, trimmed and chopped

½ cup diced onion

1 raw pickle, diced

2 TB. dulse flakes

1 TB. capers, drained

1. Combine sunflower or pumpkin seeds, lemon juice or apple cider vinegar, miso, and olive oil in a food processor and purée to a paste.

2. Add celery, onion, pickle, dulse flakes, and capers in the order listed, pulsing each ingredient a few times into mixture. Transfer to a bowl and serve immediately.

Radish and Yellow Squash Salad

This recipe is quick, simple, and really tasty. It is a great snack or side dish to complement a cooked or raw entrée. Prepare this recipe and let it sit for 15 minutes before consuming to allow the juices to come out of the radish and squash.

Yield:	Serving size:	Prep time:
1⅓ cups	About ⅔ cup	15 minutes

8 red radishes, shredded

2 medium yellow squash, shredded

Salt to taste

2 TB. goji berries

Salt to taste

1. Place radish and squash in a bowl.

2. Stir in salt and goji berries and allow to sit for 15 minutes.

FRESH FACT

Radishes come in a variety of shapes, colors, sizes, and potencies. While the red radish is the most popular, there are different varieties available for each season. Visit your local farmer's market and explore what varieties are available locally.

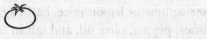

Beet and Radish Salad

Beets and radishes are root vegetables that are excellent for maintaining a healthy digestive system, liver, and kidneys. Enjoy this salad in the fall and winter to boost your immune system.

Yield:	Serving size:	Prep time:
6–8 cups	1½–2 cups	15 minutes

5 cups beet greens, torn

1 cup daikon radish, peeled and shredded

1 cup spinach or romaine lettuce

½ cup shredded beet

½ cup pumpkin seeds, soaked 1 hour and rinsed

⅓ cup sunflower seeds, soaked 1 hour and rinsed

2 tsp. lime or lemon juice

2 tsp. dried basil

1 tsp. agave, palm sugar, or honey

1 tsp. dried thyme

6–8 red radishes, sliced

Freshly ground black pepper

2 tsp. olive oil

1/4 tsp. salt

1. Put beet greens; daikon radish; spinach or lettuce; beet; pumpkin and sunflower seeds; lime or lemon juice; basil; agave, palm sugar, or honey; thyme; red radishes, pepper, olive oil, and salt in large bowl. Toss well.

Rockin' Guacamole

The addition of savory miso and tamari really make this version of everyone's favorite dip a rockin' success and is great served with crackers or lettuce leaves.

Yield:	Serving size:	Prep time:
About 1⅓ cups	About ⅔ cup	15 minutes

2 avocados, halved, seeded, scooped from outer layer, and diced

1 small onion, diced

1 medium tomato, diced

1 TB. miso

1 garlic clove, minced

2 or 3 TB. lemon or lime juice

1 or 2 tsp. tamari soy sauce

1 small jalapeno pepper, trimmed and minced, or ¼ tsp. cayenne pepper

Sea salt to taste

1. Combine avocados, onion, tomato, miso, garlic, lemon or lime juice, tamari soy sauce, hot pepper or cayenne pepper, and sea salt in a food processor and pulse to desired smoothness. Transfer to a serving bowl.

Curry Cauliflower Cous Cous

Make this recipe just once and you'll be hooked on cauliflower. The secret is to salt and squeeze the juice out of the cauliflower, which leaves you a fluffy cauliflower rice or cous cous.

Yield:	Serving size:	Prep time:
About 2⅔ cups	About ⅔ cup	30 minutes

1 head cauliflower, about 4 cups, rough chopped

½ orange bell pepper, finely diced

½ green bell pepper, finely diced

½ cup cherry tomatoes, finely diced

1 TB. curry powder (more or less to taste)

2 TB. light miso

2 tsp. cold-pressed sesame oil

½ tsp. Himalayan salt, plus more to taste

Fresh ground pepper

1. Using the s-blade in a food processor, pulse cauliflower until it resembles a rice-like consistency.

2. Transfer cauliflower to a bowl, add 1/2 teaspoon salt, and combine. Allow to sit for 15 minutes.

3. Place cauliflower mixture in a seed mylk bag and squeeze out all liquid into a bowl; reserve liquid for Creamy Cauliflower Ses'same Soup.

4. Put cauliflower "cous cous" in large bowl and add pepper, tomatoes, curry, miso, and oil and mix by hand until combined.

5. Add salt and pepper to taste.

Broccoli Rawdorf Salad

You'll love this delicious and crunchy take on traditional Waldorf salad featuring nutritious broccoli and sweet cashews.

Yield:	Serving size:	Prep time:
6 cups	2 cups	30 minutes

1 head (about 4 cups) broccoli, chopped

½ cup celery, diced

1 apple, cored and chopped

1 cup walnuts, rinsed and chopped

1 cup raisins

¼ cup red onion, diced

¾ cup cashews, soaked 1 hour, or ½ cup almond butter

¼ cup lemon juice

1 clove of garlic

2 TB. olive oil

1 TB. miso

2 tsp. mustard seed

Salt to taste

1. Place broccoli, celery, apple, walnuts, raisins, and onion in a large bowl and set aside.

2. Place cashews or almond butter, lemon juice, garlic, oil, miso, mustard seed, and salt in a blender and blend until smooth. Pour over salad ingredients in bowl and mix.

Corn 'Shroom Salad

Sweet corn and flavorful mushrooms highlight this delicious salad that's fragrant with rosemary.

Yield:	Serving size:	Prep time:
4 servings	About ⅔ cup	5 minutes

1 cup marinated mushrooms (see Chapter 10 for marinade recipes)

2 cups corn kernels, fresh or frozen and defrosted

½ cup tomato, diced

1 TB. nutritional yeast

1 tsp. fresh rosemary, minced

Sea salt to taste

Rosemary sprigs for garnish

1. Combine marinated mushrooms, corn, tomato, yeast, rosemary, and sea salt in a medium bowl and toss together gently. Garnish with rosemary sprigs and serve.

FRESH FACT

Rosemary is a perennial herb in the mint family. The plant is drought tolerant and grows well near the ocean as well as in the desert. Rosemary is high in antioxidants, iron, calcium, and vitamin B.

Avocado Apple Gadget

Amazingly healthy goji berries combine with the creaminess of avocado and the sweetness of apple for an unusually delicious salad.

Yield:	Serving size:	Prep time:
About 2 cups	About 1 cup	5 minutes

Juice of 1 orange or ½ lemon

¼ cup raisins

2 TB. goji berries

1 avocado, halved, seeded, scooped from outer skin, and diced

1 medium apple, cored and cut into matchsticks

1 TB. mesquite powder (optional)

2 tsp. cinnamon

1 tsp. maca (optional)

Pinch of sea salt

1. In a small bowl, combine orange or lemon juice with raisins and goji berries and set aside.

2. In another bowl, combine avocado, apple, mesquite powder (if using), cinnamon, maca (if using), and sea salt and mash together.

3. Stir in raisin mixture and serve.

FRESH FACT

Goji berries, also called wolfberries, have skyrocketed in popularity during the last decade and are now commonly used in beverages, teas, and desserts.

Classic Fruit Salad

The simplicity of naturally sweet fruit with a hint of cinnamon and salt is all that's needed in this healthful and hydrating salad.

Yield:	Serving size:	Prep time:
About 3 cups	About 1½ cups	20 minutes

Juice of 1 orange

2 medium apples, cored and diced

2 medium bananas, peeled and sliced

3 oranges, peeled, seeded, and segmented

2 cups red or green seedless grapes

1 cup strawberries, hulled and sliced

1 tsp. cinnamon

Pinch of sea salt

1. In a large bowl, gently toss together orange juice, apples, bananas, oranges, grapes, strawberries, cinnamon, and sea salt. Set aside for 10 minutes and serve.

Blue-Green Fruit

Spirulina provides the fabulous color for this delicious and unusual fruit salad with a hint of fresh mint.

Yield:	Serving size:	Prep time:
About 4 cups	About 1 cup	20 minutes

1 cup cubed fresh pineapple
1 cup cubed mango
1 large banana, peeled and sliced
1 cup strawberries, hulled and sliced
½ cup raisins
¼ cup goji berries
1 or 2 TB. spirulina or blue-green algae
¼ cup fresh mint leaves, finely chopped
1 tsp. cinnamon
¼ tsp. sea salt

1. In a large bowl, combine pineapple, mango, banana, strawberries, raisins, and goji berries.

2. Sprinkle in spirulina or blue-green algae, mint, cinnamon, and sea salt, toss gently to coat, and set aside to marinate for 10 minutes before serving.

Raw Entrées

In This Chapter

- Satisfying and simple selections
- Hearty wraps and rolls
- Noodling around with veggies

When hunger hits, you'll want a hearty entrée to sink your teeth into—and this chapter will provide just that. From easy-to-make wraps and rolls to stuffed veggies and even some hearty noodles, you'll find all you need to make dinner a true raw delight.

Because many of the recipes use sauces and marinades from previous pages, you'll already be well on your way to creating sensational meals beyond your culinary imagination. Be sure to keep plenty of staple ingredients on hand so they are available when needed.

These recipes will also give you a chance to utilize some interesting kitchen equipment we talked about in Chapter 7, such as the slicer and spiral thingamajig, so tie on that apron and let's get cooking—or not!

Lettuce Wraps

Wrapped-up goodness is the only way to describe these tasty delights featuring the flavor of cashews and super-nourishing sprouts.

Yield:	Serving size:	Prep time:
6 wraps	3 wraps	20 minutes

6 large romaine lettuce leaves

1 cup Cashew Cheeze (recipe in Chapter 10)

2 cups shredded carrots

2 large tomatoes, diced

1 container sprouts of your choice

1. Spread Cashew Cheeze down the center of each lettuce leaf.

2. Pile on carrots, tomatoes, and sprouts, leaving enough room for leaf to wrap around. Serve immediately.

Pesto Pepper Boats

Quick and easy, this hearty entrée makes use of raw pesto and the wonderful combination of tomato and fresh basil.

Yield:	Serving size:	Prep time:
12 pepper boats	6 pepper boats	10 minutes

1½ cups Pumpkin Seed Pesto (recipe in Chapter 10)

2 medium bell peppers, cored, seeded, and cut into 6 strips each

1 cup cherry tomatoes, halved

12 fresh basil leaves

1. Spoon pesto inside bell pepper strips. Top with tomatoes and one basil leaf on each and serve immediately.

Variation: Try using any of the other raw pesto recipes as a filling for your boats.

Marinated Veggies

This combination of vegetables is particularly tasty as a topping for pasta or simply on its own.

Yield:	Serving size:	Prep time:
About 4 cups	About 2 cups	20 minutes plus 2 hours to marinate

1 cup Orange Miso Marinade (recipe in Chapter 10)
1 cup chopped zucchini
1 cup chopped bell pepper (any color)
½ cup diced onion
1 cup mushrooms, stemmed and sliced
1 cup chopped asparagus

1. Combine Orange Miso Marinade, zucchini, bell pepper, onion, mushrooms, and asparagus in a large bowl and toss well to coat.

2. Cover tightly and transfer to the refrigerator. Allow to marinate for at least 2 hours and preferably overnight.

3. Stir well before serving.

Stuffed Portobellos

"Meaty" Portobellos are always satisfying, and in this easy recipe, a simple marinade provides a delicious savory flavor.

Yield:	Serving size:	Prep time:	Cook time:
2 mushroom caps	1 mushroom cap	20 minutes plus 2 hours to marinate	5–10 minutes

1 cup Simple Miso Marinade (recipe in Chapter 10)

2 large Portobello mushroom caps, gills removed by scraping with a spoon

1 medium sweet onion, diced

1 red bell pepper, seeded and diced

2 TB. finely chopped fresh parsley leaves

1. Place Simple Miso Marinade, mushroom caps, onion, and bell pepper in a sealable container to marinate for at least 2 hours.

2. Remove mushroom caps from marinade and then fill caps with onions and peppers from marinade.

3. Heat stuffed mushroom caps in a dehydrator for 1 hour at 115°F or in the oven for 5 to 10 minutes on the warm setting.

4. Garnish with fresh parsley and serve.

Collard Wraps

These wraps are a fun and functional way to eat raw and can be filled with any of your favorite fresh ingredients or even a spread. A dipping sauce is a nice addition.

Yield:	Serving size:	Prep time:
2 wraps	1 wrap	15 minutes

6 medium collard leaves

1 cup shredded carrots

1 cup shredded beets

1 container sprouts of your choice

1 cup spinach leaves

1 apple, cored and sliced thinly

1 recipe (about 4 TB.) Almond Miso Sauce, for dipping (recipe in Chapter 10)

1. Use a sharp knife to slice the thickness of collard leaf stems away by gliding the knife along the face and back of the leaf. The goal is to cut the stem so thinly that the leaf rolls easily.

2. Lay two leaves side by side with an inch of space between and the stems parallel. Lay a third leaf in the middle.

3. Arrange carrots, beets, sprouts, spinach, and apple along the bottom edge where the stem begins. Roll from the bottom up, tucking the edges in as you go.

4. Cut in half and serve with dipping sauce.

Variation: Try filling your wrap with Tu-No Salad, pesto, or Eggless Egg Salad.

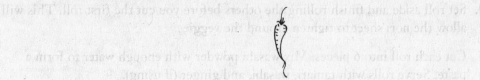

Nori Rolls

Raw nori rolls are a classic and great for creating any type of filling you like. Here, they get thinly cut vegetables with a hot wasabi kick when dipped.

Yield:	Serving size:	Prep time:
5 rolls	2½ nori rolls	15 minutes

5 raw nori sheets

1 avocado, halved, seeded, scooped from outer skin, and diced

1 medium carrot, *julienned*

1 medium celery stalk, trimmed and julienned

5 medium asparagus spears, trimmed and julienned

1 medium red bell pepper, seeded and julienned

1 container sunflower or other seed sprouts

¼ cup tamari soy sauce

¼ tsp. wasabi powder

Pickled ginger (optional)

1. Lay a nori sheet flat with the longest edge running parallel to you.

2. Arrange a thin line of avocado, carrot, celery, asparagus, pepper, and sprouts along the bottom edge, covering no more than the bottom eighth of the sheet. Let some long vegetable strips overlap the end of the sheet. Do not overstuff.

3. Put your thumbs under the bottom edge of the nori and curl your fingers around the line of veggies as you begin to roll. Roll evenly, finishing by dipping your finger in water and then running it along the final exposed strip of nori. Finish rolling after the edge has been moistened.

4. Set roll aside and finish rolling the others before you cut the first roll. This will allow the nori sheet to tighten around the veggies.

5. Cut each roll into 6 pieces. Mix wasabi powder with enough water to form a paste. Serve rolls with tamari, wasabi, and ginger (if using).

> **DEFINITION**
>
> **Julienne** is a type of cut used by chefs in which vegetables or other ingredients are cut into thin strips resembling matchsticks. Some slicing tools, such as mandolins, can create similar cuts and alleviate the careful knife work that is usually required.

Veggie Noodles and Marinara

Use a handy spiralizer to make zucchini "spaghetti" for this terrific raw copycat of pasta with sauce.

Yield:	Serving size:	Prep time:
About 4 cups	About 2 cups	25 minutes

2 medium zucchini or yellow squash, trimmed and spiralized

1 serving (about ⅓ cup) Dulse or Classic Marinara (recipe in Chapter 10)

1 serving (about 2 cups) of Marinated Veggies (recipe in Chapter 12)

1 small bell pepper, seeded and diced (any color)

1 TB. finely chopped fresh basil leaves

1. Prepare zucchini and squash "noodles" and transfer to a large mixing bowl. Lightly toss in Marinara.

2. Divide between 2 plates and top with Marinated Veggies. Garnish with bell pepper and basil.

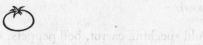

Almond Pad Thai

Kelp noodles take center stage in this terrific Thai-flavored entrée that can be made as spicy as you like.

Yield:	Serving size:	Prep time:
About 4 cups	About 2 cups	20 minutes

1 16-oz. bag kelp noodles

1 medium zucchini, trimmed and spiralized or julienned

1 medium carrot, spiralized or julienned

1 medium red bell pepper, seeded and diced

1 medium yellow bell pepper, seeded and diced

1 bunch scallions, trimmed and diced

½ cup slivered almonds

10 fresh basil leaves, preferably Thai purple basil, chopped

2 cups Almond Miso Sauce (recipe in Chapter 11)

Cayenne pepper

1. Rinse kelp noodles, squeeze out excess water, and cut. Place in a large mixing bowl.

2. Add zucchini, carrot, bell peppers, scallions, almonds, basil, and 1 cup Almond Miso Sauce to noodles, reserving some almonds and basil for garnish. Add cayenne and toss well to combine.

3. Add remaining 1 cup Almond Miso Sauce just before serving.

Raw Snacks and Desserts

In This Chapter

- Uncooked and unbelievably delicious
- Familiar flavors in a new guise
- Easy and quick sweet solutions

Desserts and snacks are still on the menu although you may be detoxifying your body, and in this chapter you'll find some amazingly delicious selections that are all raw and uncooked (despite their names). Brownies? Chocolate mousse? You won't believe your taste buds when you try these familiar and favorite flavors in a totally new guise.

Nothing here is tough to make and everything can be whipped up in virtually no time at all—so when a craving hits, you'll know you can just turn to one of these pages and happily satisfy your craving in no time! From chocolaty delights to creamy banana treats to refreshing sorbet and ice cream, it's all here just waiting to be enjoyed.

Chia Chocolate Mousse

The delicious young Thai coconut is featured in this sweet chocolaty pudding that's a real winner at dessert time.

Yield:	Serving size:	Prep time:
About 2 cups	About 1 cup	20 minutes

1 young Thai coconut, meat only

¼ cup chia gel

¼ cup coconut water

¼ cup agave nectar

3 TB. cacao powder

1 tsp. organic vanilla extract

1½ tsp. cinnamon

½ tsp. sea salt

1 TB. goji berries

1 TB. cacao nibs

1. Combine coconut, chia gel, coconut water, and agave nectar in a food processor and blend until smooth.

2. Add cacao, vanilla extract, cinnamon, and sea salt and pulse to combine.

3. Transfer to a bowl and serve sprinkled with goji berries and cacao nibs.

RAWESOME TIP

Chia gel is an indispensable creation in the raw kitchen that adds thickness and texture, not to mention omega-3, protein, fiber, and antioxidants—all without flavor that might interfere with your recipe. Make your own and keep in the refrigerator for up to one week:

Place 3 tablespoons chia seeds in a sealable jar and cover with 1½ cups water. Seal, shake, and refrigerate.

Chia in a Jar

Thick, sweet, and full of flavor, you'll love the simplicity of this treat that's similar in texture to tapioca pudding.

Yield:	Serving size:	Prep time:
About 1 cup	About ½ cup	25 minutes

3 TB. chia seeds

1 cup water

1 TB. almond butter

1 TB. agave nectar, honey, palm sugar, or equivalent amount of *stevia*

1 TB. maca

1 tsp. carob

1 tsp. cinnamon

Pinch of sea salt

1. Place chia seeds, water, almond butter, agave nectar (or other choice), and maca in a sealable jar and shake vigorously. Add the carob, cinnamon, and salt, and shake again.

2. Wait 5 minutes and shake again vigorously. After 10 minutes, shake once more. Set aside to thicken completely for another 5 minutes before serving.

DEFINITION

Stevia in its simplest form is a dried leaf from a South American plant in the mint family. It is 100 times sweeter than cane sugar, calorie-free, and low in glycemic impact, making it ideal for diabetics and dieters. Stevia comes in a variety of forms, including powdered, liquid, and even flavored—each with its own directions for use.

Stuffed Dates

The natural sweetness of dates makes them ideal for dessert making, and in this simple recipe they can be stuffed with your preferred filling and even wrapped.

Yield:	Serving size:	Prep time:
12 date halves	6 date halves	25 minutes

6 medium or large dates, halved and pitted

¼ cup coconut crème or almond butter

12 cacao beans

Sea salt to taste

Small kale or spinach leaves (optional)

1. Spoon a little coconut crème or almond butter into each date half and insert one cacao bean. Add a pinch of salt.

2. If desired, wrap each half in a spinach or kale leaf and serve.

Banana-Ginger Whip

Sweet and creamy, this pudding-like dessert with the kick of fresh ginger is great to enjoy almost anytime.

Yield:	Serving size:	Prep time:
About 2 cups	About ½ cup	10 minutes

3 medium bananas, peeled and sliced

½ cup fresh orange juice

2 TB. chia gel

2 tsp. minced fresh ginger

1 tsp. cinnamon

¼ tsp. sea salt

1. Combine bananas, orange juice, chia gel, fresh ginger, cinnamon, and sea salt in a blender and purée until smooth. Transfer to a medium bowl and serve.

Coco-Banana Gadget

This is another one of my favorite snacking recipes, which can be found in my book *Zen and the Art of Gadgeting.* The creamy delicious combination of peanut butter and bananas will make this one of your favorites, too.

Yield:	Serving size:	Prep time:
2 cups	½ cup	5 minutes

2 bananas, peeled and mashed

½ cup shredded coconut

2 TB. almond butter

2 TB. cacao nibs

2 TB. water

1 TB. mesquite powder

2 tsp. cinnamon

Pinch of salt

1. Combine bananas, coconut, almond butter, cacao nibs, water, mesquite powder, cinnamon, and salt in a large bowl.

2. Refrigerate for 1 hour and serve spoonfuls in dessert dishes.

Banana-Carob Whip

Light and sweet, this carob-flavored banana treat also provides the healthful good-ness of hemp seeds.

Yield:	Serving size:	Prep time:
About 2 cups	About ½ cup	10 minutes

3 medium bananas, peeled and sliced

½ cup water

2 TB. hemp seeds

2 TB. chia gel

1 TB. carob

2 tsp. maca

1 tsp. cinnamon

¼ tsp. sea salt

1. Combine bananas, water, hemp seeds, chia gel, carob, maca, cinnamon, and sea salt in a blender and purée until smooth. Transfer to a medium bowl and serve.

FRESH FACT

Carob is a powdered sweetener made from the seed pods of the carob tree. Carob's malty sweet taste has made it a substitute for chocolate. Other names for carob are St. John's bread and locust bean.

Superfood Truffles

You'll never find another truffle that packs as powerful a punch in the super-nutrient department as the ones in this delicious and easy recipe.

Yield:	Serving size:	Prep time:
8 to 12 truffles	2 or 3 truffles	30 minutes

8 medium or large dates, pitted

¼ cup cacao

¼ cup maca

¼ cup mesquite or carob powder

2 TB. bee pollen

2 TB. spirulina or blue-green algae

2 tsp. cinnamon

¼ tsp. sea salt

Raw honey (optional)

Cacao, maca, mesquite, or carob powder

1. Use a food processor or hand-mash together dates, cacao, maca, mesquite or carob, bee pollen, spirulina or algae, cinnamon, sea salt, and raw honey (if using). If mixture is too dry, add a drizzle of raw honey.

2. Spoon out mixture, form into 1-inch balls, and place on a plate.

3. Roll balls in cacao powder (or other choice) and serve.

FRESH FACT

Mesquite beans and leaves, from the better known mesquite wood tree used to flavor BBQ, are the primary food of coyotes in Death Valley and are extremely nutrient-rich.

Brownie Bites

As chewy and delicious as the real thing, you'll be whipping these up on a regular basis for sure.

Yield:	Serving size:	Prep time:
12 brownies	2 brownies	30 minutes

2 cups walnuts or pecans

½ cup cacao or carob

¼ cup maca

1 cup pitted dates, plus a few extra if needed

2 tsp. cinnamon

¼ tsp. sea salt

1. Combine walnuts or pecans, cacao or carob, maca, dates, cinnamon, and sea salt in a food processor and pulse to a paste. Check the consistency by squeezing mixture between your fingers. It should bind together. If too dry, add more dates.

2. Dust a small casserole dish or cookie sheet with cacao powder, then press mixture into a 6×8-inch rectangle, about 1 inch thick.

3. Cut into 12 equal pieces and serve.

Maca Macaroons

Coconut flakes and maca combine to make a delicious superfood treat. Add vanilla or cacao to the recipe to shake things up a bit. These macaroons are always a hit.

Yield:	Serving size:	Prep time:
25 macaroons	2 or 3 macaroons	30 minutes

3 cups coconut flakes

1 cup cacao powder

¼ cup agave nectar

2 TB. palm sugar

2 TB. coconut oil, melted

2 TB. maca

2 TB. ground chia

1 TB. cinnamon

2 vanilla beans, scraped, or 2 tsp. vanilla extract

⅛ tsp. salt

2 TB. water, if needed

½ cup shredded coconut, cacao powder, maca, or mesquite powder

1. In a food processor fitted with the s-blade add coconut flakes and cacao powder. Pulse to combine.

2. With the food processor running, slowly add agave nectar, palm sugar, melted coconut oil, maca, ground chia, cinnamon, vanilla, and salt.

3. Stop the food processor and check to see if the mixture will bind together when compressed; if it crumbles turn on the food processor and add water.

4. Press mixture into a tablespoon and pop out to shape or form into little balls; roll in shredded coconut (or other choice).

5. Refrigerate balls for at least 1 hour to allow the coconut oil to set. Macaroons can be stored in the refrigerator for up to 2 weeks.

Tropical Sorbet

A high-powered blender or masticating juicer will be necessary to make this amazingly refreshing treat that can be personalized according to your favorite fruits.

Yield:	Serving time:	Prep time:
About 3 cups	About ½ cup	10 minutes

1 young Thai coconut, meat and water

2½ cups frozen fruit, including mango, papaya, pineapple, or banana

1. Place coconut meat and water in the blender and begin to purée.

2. Add a little frozen fruit at a time, continuing to blend until a thick and smooth sorbet consistency is achieved.

3. Transfer to an airtight container and freeze or serve immediately.

Note: If using your juicer, be sure to use the blank plate provided with it.

RAWESOME TIP

You can make instant frozen sorbet from any frozen fruit by feeding it into your masticating juicer! The juicer should come equipped with a "blank" plate, which allows you to make nutbutters and fruit sorbets.

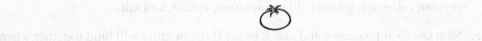

Almond-Cashew Ice Cream

You'll need an ice cream maker or masticating juicer to make this completely dairy-free ice cream that's full of nutty flavor and creamy to boot!

Yield:	Serving size:	Prep time:
About 2 cups	About ½ cup	10 minutes

½ cup almond butter

2 cups water

1 cup cashews, soaked in water for 30 minutes and drained

½ cup palm sugar or ⅓ cup agave nectar

1 TB. organic vanilla extract or 1 raw vanilla bean, split with a knife and seeds scraped from the inside

½ tsp. sea salt

1. Combine almond butter, water, cashews, palm sugar or agave nectar, vanilla extract or vanilla bean seeds, and sea salt in a blender and purée until smooth. Transfer to a clean container and cool in the freezer for 30 minutes.

2. Pour mixture into an ice cream maker and follow the manufacturer's directions. Serve immediately or freeze.

3. If using a masticating juicer, pour liquid mixture into ice cube trays and freeze.

4. Install the blank plate into the juicer and feed frozen cubes into the chute. Serve immediately or freeze.

Smoothies

In This Chapter

- Fresh and fabulous drinks
- Going green in your glass
- Magical combinations for health

If you think smoothies are simply high-sugar, frozen-fruit, and syrup creations, you're in for a surprising treat. The smoothies we are talking about contain only fresh or frozen fruit, green leafy vegetables, and magical superfoods—all things your detoxing body is craving. In this chapter, you'll be slurping some fabulous blends with interesting flavor combinations that will surely delight your taste buds and keep you on your road to health and vibrancy. When using juice or tea as a base, be sure to use only fresh-squeezed juice, such as orange juice, or one of the allowable teas, such as green or herbal.

One of the truly fun aspects of smoothie making is the room for individual creativity. The recipes in this chapter are great, but feel free to mix and match as you like. Make use of fresh, seasonal ingredients as much as you can, and don't feel restricted by specific measurements as you create. Before you know it, you'll be on your way to a magical experience. So, start your motors and let's get blending!

Apple Ginger Snap

A snap to make and delightful to drink, this smoothie gets both its color and nutrients from healthful blueberries and a bite from fresh ginger.

Yield:	Serving size:	Prep time:
2 cups	2 cups	10 minutes

1 cup water, juice, or tea

2 medium apples, cored and diced

1½ cups fresh or frozen blueberries

½ lemon, peeled and seeded

6 medium romaine lettuce leaves, chopped

1 large celery stalk, trimmed and diced (optional)

2 tsp. minced fresh ginger

1 tsp. cinnamon

Pinch of sea salt

1 TB. raw honey, palm sugar, or agave nectar (optional)

2 tsp. bee pollen (optional)

1. Combine water, apples, blueberries, lemon, lettuce leaves, celery (if using), ginger, cinnamon, sea salt, honey or other option (if using), and bee pollen (if using) in a blender and purée until smooth. Serve immediately.

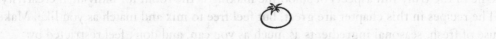

RAWESOME TIP

If you aren't using a high-powered blender, you may need to thoroughly cut up the fruits and leafy greens and pre-blend tough items in the water, juice, or tea you are using initially. This will extend the life of your blender and help make a smoother smoothie.

Green Machine

Gorgeous and green, this smoothie provides some excellent fruit antioxidants as well as powerful spirulina.

Yield:	Serving size:	Prep time:
2 cups	2 cups	10 minutes

1½ cups water, juice, or tea

1½ medium apples, cored and diced

1½ medium oranges, peeled and seeded

1 handful fresh spinach leaves

1½ TB. spirulina or blue-green algae

1 TB. chia seeds

2 tsp. minced fresh ginger

1 tsp. cinnamon

Pinch of sea salt

1. Combine water, apples, oranges, spinach, spirulina, chia seeds, ginger, cinnamon, and sea salt in a blender and purée until smooth. Serve immediately.

RAWESOME TIP

Don't ever feel like you have to finish your smoothie in one sitting if you can't, especially at the beginning of your detox. Put the leftovers in a sealable jar and save it for later or refrigerate overnight.

Banana Orange Kale

This terrific, simple combination will surprise you with its wonderfully sweet flavor and creamy consistency.

Yield:	Serving size:	Prep time:
2½ cups	2½ cups	10 minutes

2 cups water, juice, or tea
1½ medium bananas, peeled and sliced
1 medium orange, peeled and seeded
4 medium kale leaves, stemmed and chopped
1 tsp. cinnamon
Pinch of sea salt

1. Combine water, bananas, orange, kale leaves, cinnamon, and sea salt in a blender and purée until smooth. Serve immediately.

RAWESOME TIP

Using frozen pieces of fresh fruit you've prepared ahead of time in your smoothies will make for a thicker and colder result.

Monkey King

Banana and cacao are the featured flavors in this delicious smoothie that's guaranteed to become a true favorite.

Yield:	Serving size:	Prep time:
2 cups	2 cups	5 minutes

1½ cups water, juice, or tea
2 medium bananas, peeled and sliced
1 TB. almond butter
1 TB. spirulina or blue-green algae (optional)
2 tsp. cacao
2 tsp. mesquite powder
1½ tsp. maca
1½ tsp. carob
1 tsp. cinnamon
Pinch of sea salt

1. Combine water, bananas, almond butter, spirulina or algae (if using), cacao, mesquite, maca, carob, cinnamon, and sea salt in a blender and purée until smooth. Serve immediately.

Berry Best

Blueberries combine with two newer kids on the block—açai and goji berries—in this great-tasting smoothie that also features healthful aloe vera.

Yield:	Serving size:	Prep time:
About 2 cups	About 2 cups	10 minutes

1½ cups water, juice, or tea

2 cups fresh or frozen blueberries

¼ to ½ cup aloe vera, fresh and peeled or juice

½ lemon, peeled and seeded

2 TB. açai, frozen, juice, or powder

2 TB. goji berries, presoaked in water for 1 hour

1 TB. maca

1 TB. spirulina or blue-green algae

1½ tsp. minced fresh ginger

2 tsp. chia seeds

Pinch of sea salt

1. Combine water, blueberries, aloe vera, lemon, açai, goji berries, maca, spirulina or algae, ginger, chia seeds, and sea salt in a blender and purée until smooth. Serve immediately.

FRESH FACT

Aloe vera juice is a popular drink in the Hispanic culture and is often taken to relieve indigestion.

Hemp Seed Supreme

Packed full of goodness your body will appreciate, this smoothie gets its creaminess from bananas and a further layer of flavor from cacao and cinnamon.

Yield:	Serving size:	Prep time:
About 1½ cups	About 1½ cups	10 minutes

1½ cups water, juice, or tea
1½ medium bananas, peeled and sliced
2 TB. hemp seeds
2 TB. mesquite powder
1 TB. maca
1 TB. spirulina
1 TB. chia
1 TB. bee pollen
1 TB. cacao
1 tsp. cinnamon
Pinch of sea salt

1. Combine water, bananas, hemp seeds, mesquite powder, maca, spirulina, chia, bee pollen, cacao, cinnamon, and sea salt in a blender and purée until smooth. Serve immediately.

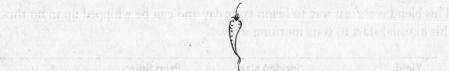

Coconut Cooler

Tasty coconut and bananas come together in this satisfying and refreshing smoothie that's great for any time of day.

Yield:	Serving size:	Prep time:
About 2 cups	About 2 cups	20 minutes

1 young Thai coconut, meat and water

1½ medium bananas, peeled and sliced

1 TB. cacao

1 TB. maca

1 TB. spirulina or blue-green algae (optional)

1 TB. chia seeds

1 tsp. cinnamon

Pinch of sea salt

1. Combine coconut, bananas, cacao, maca, spirulina or algae (if using), chia seeds, cinnamon, and sea salt in a blender and purée until smooth. Serve immediately.

Miso Sunrise

This blend is a great way to begin your day and can be whipped up in no time. Give this unusual start to your morning a try.

Yield:	Serving size:	Prep time:
1½ cups	1½ cups	2 minutes

1½ cups warm water

2 TB. miso

1 TB. fresh lemon or orange juice

2 tsp. minced fresh ginger

¼ tsp. cayenne pepper, or to taste

1. Combine water, miso, lemon juice, ginger, and cayenne pepper in a blender and pulse several times to blend. Pour into a mug or bowl and serve immediately.

FRESH FACT

In Japan, almost everyone starts their day with a morning cup of miso—a tasty and healthful alternative to coffee. Give it a try and see whether it quickly becomes a healthful habit for you, too.

Citrus Flush

This recipe is great for liver support and can be enjoyed any time you like. Read more about this type of flush in Dr. Rudolph Stone's *Purifying Diet* (see Resources).

Yield:	Serving size:	Prep time:
2 cups	2 cups	5 minutes

2 cups fresh-squeezed orange or grapefruit juice

Juice of ½ lemon or lime

1½ TB. olive oil

1 large garlic clove, minced

Pinch of cayenne pepper

1. Combine orange or grapefruit juice, lemon juice, olive oil, garlic, and cayenne pepper in a blender and pulse until smooth. Serve immediately.

RAWESOME TIP

Chewing fresh parsley after consuming garlic will help remove the taste and smell from your mouth.

Mango-Basil Bliss

Sweet and delicious mango combines with strawberries and spinach for an unusual combination with a hint of fragrant basil.

Yield:	Serving size:	Prep time:
About 2 cups	About 1 cup	10 minutes

2 mangos, peeled, seeded, and diced

1 cup strawberries, hulled and sliced

2 cups fresh spinach leaves, firmly packed and chopped

1 cup water or ice

½ cup fresh basil leaves, firmly packed and chopped

1½ tsp. minced fresh ginger

1 tsp. cinnamon

Pinch of sea salt

1. Combine mangos, strawberries, spinach, water, basil, ginger, cinnamon, and sea salt in a blender and purée until smooth. Serve immediately.

Strawberry Coconut Smoothie

Pink, smooth, and delicious; this smoothie is a creamy tasty treat that can be enjoyed any time of the day.

Yield:	Serving size:	Prep time:
About 4 cups	About 2 cups	10 minutes

1 young Thai coconut, water and meat

1 cup strawberries, fresh or frozen

½ banana

¼ cup hemp seeds

2 TB. lucuma (optional)

1 TB. cacao powder (optional)

1 tsp. cinnamon

Pinch of sea salt

Agave nectar, stevia, or palm sugar (optional)

1. Combine coconut, strawberries, banana, hemp seeds, lucuma (if using), cacao powder (if using), cinnamon, and sea salt in a blender and purée until smooth. Sweeten with agave nectar (or other choice) if necessary. Serve immediately.

 RAWESOME TIP

The green tops on strawberries are edible and are actually good for your teeth. Consume only the tops of fresh strawberries that are chemical free or organic. One of the best ways to get your strawberry greens is to blend them into your smoothie.

Juices

In This Chapter

- Carrot juice combos that rock
- Refreshing juices for hydration
- Marvelous medleys of flavor

Fiber is critical for proper digestion and elimination. The body prefers the plant fiber in raw foods. There are times, however, when fiber can be a burden on the system and you may need to give your body a break. But how do you eat celery without eating the fiber? You juice it!

Juicing is a phenomenal way to detox and heal the body. Countless authors and health practitioners extol the benefits of separating the fresh, nutrient-rich juice in fruits, vegetables, roots, and herbs from their inherent plant fiber. In this way, you'll receive vital nourishment and hydration without taxing the digestive system. That means the stomach, liver, pancreas, gall bladder, and intestines get a vacation. Just the kidneys are still working, filtering the juice and eliminating toxins.

You don't need to engage in a juice fast to experience the hydrating and energy-boosting power of juice. Everyone can benefit from enjoying juice before a meal, as a snack, or in place of a meal. Keep in mind the important food-combining principles we discussed in Chapter 3, however, and drink juices before meals to prevent digestive traffic jams.

Str8 Carrot

This is a great base recipe for carrot juicing. The ginger and lemon add a nice zing and balance the sweetness of the carrots.

Yield:	Serving size:	Prep time:
4 cups	2 cups	10 minutes

8 medium carrots
1 one-inch piece fresh ginger
½ lemon
About 1 cup purified water

1. Prepare carrots, ginger, and lemon according to juicer manufacturer's recommendations.

2. Put carrots, ginger, and lemon through the juicer and use water to thin, as desired, before drinking.

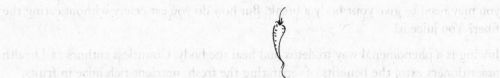

RAWESOME TIP

Adding water to fresh carrot juice and its blends reduces the dramatic effect large quantities of carrots may have on blood sugar (particularly for those who are diabetic) while also reducing the intense sweetness.

Carrot Spinach

Powerfully nutritious spinach combines with sweet carrots for another great juice base in your juicing repertoire.

Yield:	Serving size:	Prep time:
4 cups	2 cups	10 minutes

6 medium carrots
4 cups fresh spinach leaves, packed
About 1 cup purified water

1. Prepare carrots according to the juicer manufacturer's recommendations. Wash spinach leaves to remove all grit and dirt.

2. Put carrots and spinach through the juicer and use water to thin, as desired, before drinking.

DETOXER'S ALERT

Consuming large quantities of carrots or carrot juice can cause your skin to appear orange. This temporary change is not cause for concern and usually dissipates within a short time.

Apple Carrot

This delicious combination results in a sweet and zesty juice that can be made "fruitier" by adding more apples.

Yield:	Serving size:	Prep time:
4 cups	2 cups	10 minutes

8 medium carrots

1 medium apple

1 one-inch piece fresh ginger

½ lemon

About 1 cup purified water

1. Prepare carrots, apple, ginger, and lemon according to the juicer manufacturer's recommendations.

2. Put carrots, apple, ginger, and lemon through the juicer and use water to thin, as desired, before drinking.

FRESH FACT

Fresh, unpasteurized carrot juice is the highest source of vitamin A compared to all other foods and a rich source of vitamins C, D, E, G, and K. It has been shown to balance the entire body, encourage appetite, and support healthy digestion.

Carrot Fennel

Fennel adds a delightful licorice flavor to this carrot blend that also features tangy ginger and refreshing celery.

Yield:	Serving size:	Prep time:
4 cups	2 cups	10 minutes

5 medium carrots

4 medium celery stalks

½ medium fennel bulb, with or without fronds

1 one-inch piece fresh ginger

About 1 cup purified water

1. Prepare carrots, celery, fennel, and ginger according to the juicer manufacturer's recommendations.

2. Put carrots, celery, fennel, and ginger through the juicer and use water to thin, as desired, before drinking.

FRESH FACT

Delicious fennel boasts an unusual phytonutrient compound called anethole, the primary component of its oil. Studies have repeatedly shown anethole's anti-inflammatory capability as well as its anti-cancer effect.

4 by 4

This standard carrot and celery combination is good for beginning juicers and can be enhanced with any number of veggies or fruit, including the snappy parsley used here. Try adding citrus fruit or even other fresh herbs.

Yield:	Serving size:	Prep time:
4 cups	2 cups	10 minutes

4 medium carrots
4 medium celery stalks
Small bunch parsley
About 1 cup purified water

1. Prepare carrots, celery, and parsley according to the juicer manufacturer's recommendations.

2. Put carrots, celery, and parsley through the juicer and use water to thin, as desired, before drinking.

FRESH FACT

Parsley is the world's most popular herb and gets its name from the Greek word meaning "rock celery" (parsley is a relative of celery). It is a biennial plant and extremely easy to grow for the home gardener.

Carrot, Lettuce, and Kale

Although maybe an odd idea at first, juicing lettuces and leafy greens can give you terrific access to their amazing nutrients without filling up on fiber. Combined with carrots and ginger, the flavor is terrific.

Yield:	Serving size:	Prep time:
4 cups	2 cups	10 minutes

4 medium carrots
½ head lettuce, any type
3 large kale leaves
1 one-inch piece fresh ginger
About 1 cup purified water

1. Prepare carrots, lettuce, kale, and ginger according to the juicer manufacturer's recommendations.

2. Put carrots, lettuce, kale, and ginger through the juicer and use water to thin, as desired, before drinking.

 RAWESOME TIP

Refrain from washing lettuce and leafy greens until just before eating or juicing, because water can leech out vital nutrients and wither their hearty crispness.

Juice Medley

Variety is the spice of life—as is a dose of pungent garlic in this fabulous juice full of vital nutrients.

Yield:	Serving size:	Prep time:
4 cups	2 cups	10 minutes

1 medium apple

4 medium celery stalks

2 medium carrots

2 cups broccoli florets

1 medium garlic clove

About 1 cup purified water

1. Prepare apple, celery, carrots, broccoli, and garlic according to the juicer manufacturer's recommendations.

2. Put apple, celery, carrots, broccoli, and garlic through the juicer and use water to thin, as desired, before drinking.

RAWESOME TIP

Broccoli stalks are equally flavorful as the darker-green florets. The stalks can be used in a variety of raw recipes, such as salads, soups, and juices—so don't discard when trimming.

Tree of Life

Cucumbers are great for skin, hair, and nails and are a great source of mineral-rich hydration. Here, they team up with other refreshing and flavorful vegetables for a delicious and thirst-quenching drink.

Yield:	Serving size:	Prep time:
4 cups	2 cups	10 minutes

2 medium cucumbers

3 medium celery stalks

4 medium kale leaves

¼ bunch parsley

1 small garlic clove

½ lemon

1. Prepare cucumbers, celery, kale, parsley, garlic, and lemon according to the juicer manufacturer's recommendations.

2. Put cucumbers, celery, kale, parsley, garlic, and lemon through the juicer and drink immediately.

FRESH FACT

Cucumbers are nearly 95 percent water and require no thinning when juiced. Their skins are an excellent source of silica, potassium, and magnesium, so look for organic cukes—and don't peel them before juicing.

Cucumber Cilantro

Cool and tasty with your own level of "kick," this delicious juice is both refreshing and rejuvenating.

Yield:	Serving size:	Prep time:
4 cups	2 cups	10 minutes

1 medium cucumber

3 medium celery stalks

1 medium apple

¼ bunch cilantro

1 one-inch piece fresh ginger

½ lime

1 small Jalapeño pepper or cayenne pepper

1. Prepare cucumber, celery, apple, cilantro, ginger, lime, and pepper according to the juicer manufacturer's recommendations.

2. Put cucumber, celery, apple, cilantro, ginger, and lime through the juicer and drink immediately.

DETOXER'S ALERT

When handling jalapeño peppers (and any other fresh hot peppers), remember to wash your hands before touching your eyes or face to prevent a burning sensation. Be sure to clean cutting boards as well.

Three "C"s, One "G"

Just plain delicious is the way to describe this combo that's great to sip or gulp.

Yield:	Serving size:	Prep time:
4 cups	2 cups	10 minutes

1 medium cucumber
2 medium celery stalks
2 medium carrots
1 one-inch piece fresh ginger

1. Prepare cucumber, celery, carrots, and ginger according to the juicer manufacturer's recommendations.

2. Put cucumber, celery, carrots, and ginger through the juicer and drink immediately.

FRESH FACT

Did you know juices and the art of juicing can be traced to biblical times and are recommended by the Essenes in the Dead Sea Scrolls as a healing method?

CAB

This drink is the perfect nutritional taxi ride for finding plenty of super healthy *betalains* and other phytonutrients.

Yield:	Serving size:	Prep time:
4 cups	2 cups	10 minutes

2 medium cucumbers

1 medium apple

2 cups roughly chopped beets

1 one-inch piece fresh ginger

1. Prepare cucumbers, apple, beets, and ginger according to the juicer manufacturer's recommendations.

2. Put cucumbers, apple, beets, and ginger through the juicer and drink immediately.

DEFINITION

Betalains, found most commonly in beets, are healthy phytonutrients. Betanin and vulgaxanthin are the two best-studied betalains found in beets, and both have been shown to provide antioxidant, anti-inflammatory, and detoxification support.

Ring My Bell

Naturally sweet bell peppers star in this delicious juice combination that can be made lively and tangy as well, depending on the level of "hot" you choose.

Yield:	Serving size:	Prep time:
4 cups	2 cups	10 minutes

2 bell peppers, red, orange, or yellow

2 medium carrots

2 medium cucumbers

4 medium kale leaves

2 cups spinach

1 small jalapeño pepper, seeded, or more to taste

Handful of cilantro and/or parsley

1. Prepare bell peppers, carrots, cucumbers, kale, spinach, jalapeño pepper, and cilantro or parsley according to the juicer manufacturer's recommendations.

2. Put bell peppers, carrots, cucumbers, kale, spinach, jalapeño pepper, and cilantro or parsley through the juicer and drink immediately.

 RAWESOME TIP

Removing the seeds from a jalapeño pepper greatly reduces its "heat" because most of its powerful zing is located there.

Virgin Mary

You'll never go back to bottled or canned tomato juice after this amazingly flavorful version that's super easy to make.

Yield:	Serving size:	Prep time:
4 cups	2 cups	10 minutes

3 medium tomatoes
3 medium celery stalks
1 cup parsley
1 medium garlic clove
½ tsp. sea salt
⅛ tsp. freshly ground black pepper

1. Prepare tomatoes, celery, parsley, and garlic, according to the juicer manufacturer's recommendations.

2. Put tomatoes, celery, parsley, garlic, salt, and pepper through the juicer and drink immediately.

Creating your own juice blends can be easy and tasty. The best way is to start with a mild base and expand from there, incorporating stronger ingredients.

Mild	Medium	Strong	Look Out!
Aloe vera	Beets	Citrus peel	Horseradish
Coconut water	Broccoli	Garlic	Hot peppers
Cucumber	Burdock	Ginger	
Lettuce	Carrots	Lemons	
Spinach	Cauliflower	Limes	
	Collard greens	Mustard greens	
	Grapefruit	Radishes	
	Green onions	Onions	
	Green herbs	Turmeric	
	Kale		
	Most fruits		
	Oranges		
	Sprouts		

Consider adopting fresh juices into your weekly and daily schedule. Juicing is an ideal way to get hydration and nutrition in a fresh and tasty form.

Let Raw Food Be Thy Medicine

Part

4

What is it about raw food and the wondrous other living foods that can make such a difference in our health? In this part, you'll learn about the nutritional aspects of many of the foods you are eating as well as have your questions answered about calorie intake and other issues. You'll gain great respect and knowledge when it comes to healing foods—particularly those that have super-powerful nutrition—and learn about other practices such as sprouting. Finally, you'll become familiar with the buzzwords "prebiotics" and "probiotics" and understand the tremendous health values of eating fermented and cultured foods.

Raw Food and Your Nutritional Needs

In This Chapter

- Answers about calorie and protein concerns
- Understanding macro- and micro-nutrients
- Taking advantage of antioxidants and fiber

When embarking on any type of new eating program, most people have concerns about whether or not their nutritional needs will be met. And in the case of beginning a raw food detoxification regimen, there are certainly a number of questions that arise.

In this chapter, we answer them all, from whether or not you can get enough calories and protein to important distinctions between carbohydrates and fats found in the plant world as opposed to the animal world. By the end of the discussion, all your concerns will surely be addressed, and you'll be more convinced than ever that a raw food detox is the way to go for optimal nutrition, health, and overall wellness.

The Question of Calories

Calories are units of energy present in foods—the fuel factor. Carbohydrates, fats, and protein all contain calories, but there is more to food and life than just calories. Water doesn't have any calories, yet we can't live without it. Vitamins, minerals, and antioxidants don't necessarily have caloric counts, yet they are vital for life.

So how important is it to know the number of calories you are taking in? A person who is counting calories is usually looking to lose weight or is involved in athletic training. Calories are only part of the health equation, however, and by focusing solely on calories, vital nutrients can be overlooked. The focus should be on the quality of the calories we choose to consume. Are we consuming "questionable calories," also known as empty calories, found in most processed foods? Counting calories becomes unnecessary when you consume only the nutrient-dense, hydrating, and fresh foods called for on the raw detox programs. As long as a balance is maintained between the three types of foods—carbohydrates, fats, and proteins—then the calorie issue balances itself.

Less Is More

In actuality, the consumption of too much food (meaning too many calories) may actually shorten your life. Although eating and digesting food provides nourishment for the body, it also causes oxidative stress—especially when eating is done in excess of the body's needs. It's kind of like filling your car's gas tank beyond its capacity. Gasoline ends up spilling, causing waste and becoming a toxic hazard. Calorie restriction as a practice has been proven effective in increasing life span and minimizing the effects of aging in studies conducted on yeast, fish, mice, rats, and dogs. By analyzing the diets of the longest-living cultures, we see the positive benefits of calorie restriction.

 FRESH FACT

The concept of "calorie restriction" was discovered in 1934, when Cornell University professors found that feeding laboratory rats a nutritionally complete, yet calorically restricted, diet extended their lives and reduced signs of aging. Since then, people around the globe have adopted this way of eating to ensure personal health and longevity.

Here are some benefits of taking in less than 10 percent to 25 percent of the average calorie intake of the general U.S. population:

- Lower LDL (bad cholesterol)
- Higher HDL (good cholesterol)
- Lower BMI (body mass index)
- Lower triglycerides
- Lower blood pressure

- Lower insulin levels
- Reduced inflammation
- Improved memory

Don't Count on Them for Now

With raw food detox, we don't bother counting calories. The focus is on quality, and we allow quantity to work itself out. When you exchange low-quality, empty-calorie, processed foods for high-quality, nutrient-dense, raw foods, you inevitably end up eating less and being more satisfied. This is a result of fiber content and volume satiety (among other things). With this way of eating, you naturally end up consuming fewer calories without even trying.

DETOXER'S ALERT

In many cases, dehydration —or the body's need for water—is misinterpreted as hunger. When you feel hungry, first reach for a glass of water and then consider eating hydrating, nutrient-dense foods such as fresh fruit. If hunger persists, it may be time to eat something denser, such as an avocado, a raw energy bar, or trail mix. If it's mealtime, then hunker down to a hearty raw meal.

Weight Loss

You can lose weight quickly with a raw food detox, especially when combined with juicing and fasting. During a fast and cleanse, I've seen people lose a pound a day throughout the fast. They'll often continue to lose weight after the fast has been broken if they continue eating raw foods. By no means are these people wasting away or starving themselves. Caloric and nutrient intake is always at healthy levels during the raw food detox programs included in this book—the only difference is that the calories and nutrients are fresh, uncooked, and unprocessed.

Dramatic weight loss often tapers off over time and eventually plateaus due to water weight being shed. Retaining water weight can be a defense mechanism the body uses to buffer acidic pH and toxins in the body. Once toxins have been removed and body pH has been normalized, the body releases water weight, and allows for fresh rehydration. To continue losing weight at this point, it may be necessary to engage in cardiovascular exercise—and rebounding is the safest, easiest, and most accessible type of cardio you can do. The body may need a break as well. There are countless intricate processes going on behind the scenes in our bodies. With dramatic weight loss, the body may need time to adjust its metabolism, rebuild organs, and tighten up support systems before it can shed more weight. If you are stuck at a plateau, you can scale back to a highly raw diet (60 percent–80 percent raw) until you feel comfortable engaging in another round of raw food detox.

Carbohydrates

Carbohydrates are calorie-rich foods that get you where you need to go. There are essentially two types of natural carbohydrates—simple and complex—and a third "unnatural" type: refined. Briefly stated, there are simple carbohydrates such as fruits; complex carbohydrates such as root vegetables, grains, and corn; and refined carbohydrates such as white sugar and corn syrup. These refined carbohydrate foods contain empty calories and are known as junk food. Refined sugars are unnatural, processed carbohydrate impostors that have been stripped of all their beneficial qualities.

Low or no quality equals dangerous to your body and its long-term health. White flour and white rice are examples. They are nutritionally deficient and unbalanced. Taking in these foods throws off the balance of the body, so beware.

Simple Sugars

The calories in simple carbohydrates consist of simple sugars, which easily turn into energy. Nature gives us a signal when foods are calorie-rich, simple carbohydrates: they're usually vibrantly colored and sweet. Fruits are the most readily available form of raw food carbohydrates, and the body can easily digest them in the shortest period of time of all the foods we consume. They give us a burst of energy to function in a fast-paced world.

Melons are the quickest to digest of just about all the sweet fruits. Because of this, they should be eaten first and separately from all other types of food. When I enjoy melons, I sprinkle Himalayan or sea salt on top to get a salty-sweet experience.

Here are the digestive transit times of fruit and vegetables:

- Melons: 15–30 minutes
- Sweet fruits, such as figs: 30–45 minutes
- Semi-acidic fruits, such as berries: 1–1½ hours
- Acidic fruits, such as oranges: 1½–2 hours
- Non-sweet fruits and vegetables: 2–3 hours

Complex Carbs

Complex carbohydrates are sometimes referred to as starches. They consist of many simple carbohydrates bound together in a molecular chain. Complex carbohydrates in the living world represent structural and storage components in organisms. In plants, starch is the complex carbohydrate whose purpose is storing sugars. In animals, it is represented as glycogen, which is made up of chains of simple carbohydrates (sugars) that can be easily converted into energy.

The starches most people are familiar with are breads, pastas, beans, rice, potatoes, carrots, beets, and corn. In the raw food detox program complex carbohydrates are avoided because they're too complex for quick digestion. The process of breaking down complex carbohydrates into simple sugars takes energy, and that's energy that can be used for other metabolic processes in the body, such as detoxification.

Most starches are actually inedible in their raw forms. Grains, rice, potatoes, and beans shouldn't be eaten raw. There are a few exceptions, including corn, green beans and peas, carrots, and beets. Grains can be sprouted and consumed, but their nutritional profile is so poor that it often isn't worth the trouble. Quinoa is one of the few exceptions in the world of grains, and it is also gluten-free—making it a safe choice for those with a gluten intolerance (an inability to digest specific substances found in wheat).

RAWESOME TIP

Symptoms of gluten intolerance include the following:

- Constipation
- Diarrhea
- Skin rash
- Flatulence, bloating, and gas pain
- Joint pain
- Fatigue
- Headache

Proteins

If I were given one goji berry for every person who asked me, "Where do you get your protein?", I'd have a lot of goji berries. And yes, I get some of my protein from goji berries. All raw foods contain a percentage of each of the three macro-nutrients—protein, fat, and carbohydrates. Foods that are protein dominant (greater than 33 percent) are proteins, fat-dominant foods are called fats, and carbohydrate-dominant foods are considered carbohydrates. By this definition, many of the foods that people consider "protein foods" can actually be both fat- and protein-dominant. For example, beef is very high in protein, but unfortunately it is also quite high in saturated fat.

Actual Needs

To get to the bottom of this protein question, we need to determine what percentage of protein in the diet is ideal for health. Because we know that carbohydrates and fats supply the body with needed energy, what does protein do? Proteins are building blocks made up of smaller units called amino acids. How much building and tearing down gets done in your adult years? This answer depends on your level of activity as well as other lifestyle factors, like stress and the amount of toxins you may consume.

Mother's milk is around 6 percent protein. If 6 percent protein is good enough for a growing baby, it should be enough for adults. The standard American diet weighs in at around 16 percent protein, according to calculations done by Dr. Douglas N. Graham in his book *The 80/10/10 Diet*. This percentage includes cooked protein, of which a portion is unusable. Most people are surprised at this number, thinking they're eating more protein than that—but actually, their protein foods are more accurately described as fat-dominant. By eating a variety of raw foods and focusing on getting a majority of your calories from fresh fruits and vegetables, you can easily get more than 6 percent of your calories from protein. Add an avocado and a handful of nuts or seeds into your daily intake, and all your bases are covered.

Amino Acids

As we mentioned earlier, some amount of protein exists in all raw foods because they contain amino acids. A total of 22 amino acids are standard in living organisms. These amino acids are the building blocks used by the body to form protein, and each of the 22 amino acids connects with other amino acids in a multitude of combi-nations to form our bodies.

You'll be happy to know that you don't need to consume all your amino acids in one sitting to use them. The body can utilize and store amino acids provided in various meals throughout the day. At one time, common belief was that complete proteins had to be constructed at every meal, which led to people striving to combine rice and beans or any other variety of complete protein combos. We know now that this is not necessary. Respecting the laws of food combining, though, is still necessary for proper digestion, so keep those proteins and starches in separate meals and be mindful of digestion times.

Ideal Sources

When eating a variety of fresh, raw foods, you are almost assured of meeting all your protein needs. In actuality, a number of raw foods are raw-protein superstars. Hemp seeds, spirulina, bee pollen, and chia seeds are four high-quality sources of complete protein. As for fresh produce protein content, broccoli is made up of 20 percent protein, peas are 23 percent, asparagus is 27 percent, and spinach is 30 percent. Mushrooms, such as portobello, cremini, and shiitake, also have high protein contents. Rest assured that the protein found in raw and living foods is beyond most everyone's daily needs and is of the highest quality.

The following chart lists the macronutrient and calorie content of a small collection of fruits, vegetables, and fats, as well as a few starches and grains commonly eaten among raw fooders.

Included in the chart are:

- Calories
- Grams of water and fiber
- Percentage of calories from carbohydrates, protein, and fat
- Grams of carbohydrates, protein, and fat

All food items are listed in 100-gram (3.5-ounce) portions—the size of a small 6-inch banana, a small 2.5-inch apple, or 2.5 medium stalks of celery. The information in these charts is derived from the USDA National Nutrient Database for Standard Reference, Release 18, available online at www.nal.usda.gov/fnic/foodcomp/Data, and was compiled by Laurie Masters for the book *80/10/10 Diet* by Doug Graham and is reprinted by permission.

Fruits	Cal 100g	Water grams	Fiber grams	Carb % Cal	Pro % Cal	Fat % Cal	Carb grams	Pro grams	Fat grams
APPLES	52	86	2	95%	2%	3%	13.8	0.3	0.2
BANANAS	89	75	3	93%	4%	3%	22.8	1.1	0.3
BLACKBERRIES	43	88	5	79%	11%	10%	9.6	1.4	0.5
DATES (medjool)	277	21	7	97%	2%	1%	75.0	1.8	0.2
FIGS	74	79	3	93%	4%	3%	19.2	0.8	0.3
GRAPES	69	81	1	95%	3%	2%	18.1	0.7	0.2
MANGOS	65	82	2	93%	3%	4%	17.0	0.5	0.3
NECTARINES	44	88	2	86%	8%	6%	10.6	1.1	0.3
ORANGES, CA (Valencia)	49	86	3	88%	7%	5%	11.9	1.0	0.3
PEACHES	39	89	2	86%	8%	6%	9.5	0.9	0.3
PEARS	58	84	3	97%	2%	1%	15.5	0.4	0.1
STRAWBERRIES	32	91	2	85%	7%	8%	7.7	0.7	0.3
WATERMELON	30	91	0	87%	7%	6%	7.6	0.6	0.2

Vegetables									
BROCCOLI	34	89	3	70%	20%	10%	7.6	2.8	0.4
CABBAGE	24	92	2	83%	14%	3%	5.6	1.4	0.1
CARROTS	41	88	3	90%	6%	4%	9.6	0.9	0.2
CAULIFLOWER	25	92	3	77%	20%	3%	5.3	2.0	0.1
CELERY	14	95	2	76%	12%	13%	3.0	0.7	0.2
KALE	50	84	2	72%	16%	12%	10.0	3.3	0.7
LETTUCE (romaine)	17	95	2	68%	17%	15%	3.3	1.2	0.3
SPINACH	23	91	2	54%	31%	15%	3.6	2.9	0.4
Vegetable Fruits (nonsweet fruits)									
CUCUMBER	15	95	1	84%	10%	6%	3.6	0.6	0.1
TOMATOES, RED	18	95	1	79%	12%	9%	3.9	0.9	0.2
ZUCCHINI	16	95	7	72%	18%	10%	3.3	1.2	0.2
Starches & Grains (only very young, sweet peas/corn recommended)									
BUCKWHEAT	343	10	10	79%	13%	8%	71.5	13.3	3.4
CHICKPEAS (garbanzo beans)	364	12	17	68%	18%	14%	60.7	19.3	6.0
CORN	86	76	3	78%	10%	12%	19.0	3.2	1.2
PEAS, EDIBLE PODDED	42	89	3	73%	23%	4%	7.6	2.8	1.2
SWEET POTATO	86	77	3	94%	5%	1%	20.1	1.6	0.1
WHEAT (soft red winter)	331	12	13	85%	11%	4%	74.2	10.4	1.6
WILD RICE	357	8	6	82%	15%	3%	74.9	14.7	1.1

Fats									
ALMONDS	578	5	12	14%	13%	3%	19.7	21.3	50.6
AVOCADOS (California)	167	72	7	19%	4%	77%	8.6	2.0	15.4
CASHEWS	553	5	3	23%	11%	66%	30.2	18.2	43.8
COCONUT MEAT (mature)	354	47	9	18%	3%	79%	15.2	3.3	33.5
FLAXSEEDS	492	9	28	28%	14%	58%	34.3	19.5	34.0
HEMP SEEDS	533	-	3	17%	27%	56%	23.0	37.0	33.0
MACADAMIA NUTS	718	1	9	18%	4%	88%	13.8	7.9	75.8
OLIVES, CANNED (small to x-large)	115	80	3	20%	2%	78%	6.3	0.8	10.7
PINE NUTS	673	2	4	8%	7%	85%	13.1	13.7	68.4
WALNUTS (English)	654	4	7	9%	8%	83%	13.7	15.2	65.2
SESAME SEEDS	573	5	12	6%	11%	73%	23.5	17.7	49.7
SUNFLOWER SEEDS	570	5	11	13%	14%	73%	18.8	22.8	49.6
OIL (all types)	884	0	0	0%	0%	100%	0	0	100

Fats

Fat phobia is a common trend today due to media hype and a vague understanding of the types of fats and their purposes.

Unfortunately, fats have been unjustly demonized in the world of health. Yes, there are some "bad" fats out there—but not all fats are the enemy. Cooked fats and fats from animal sources are the troublemakers. The fats of the plant world are what we want for raw food detox and health. These fats are cholesterol free and typically contain the balance of fats the body needs. They help lubricate, insulate, and moisturize the body and even stabilize mood.

Not only do fats have the capability to insulate you from the cold, but they also bind with environmental toxins. Raw plant fats also contain the fat-splitting enzyme lipase, which can help dissolve old, inferior fat deposits in the body in exchange for superior plant-based fats. Eating healthful fats can help eliminate stored unhealthy fat from the body. In cases of obesity, many individuals are deficient in lipase production. Raw plant fats bring in the lipase needed to metabolize those stubborn fat deposits.

Healthy Unsaturated Fats

Unsaturated and saturated are the two classes of fats most people know. Unsaturated fats are separated further into two classes: monounsaturated or polyunsaturated. The distinction between these fats involves their chemical structures. Most plants contain a portion of each of these unsaturated fats, with one of the fats being dominant.

One type of polyunsaturated fat is known as an essential fatty acid (EFA). EFAs are found in high concentrations in the brain, and deficiencies have been associated with neurological degeneration. The body must consume EFAs in the form of food or supplements. These essentials are linoleic (omega-6) and linolenic (omega-3) fatty acids and are present in most raw foods in some amount. Specific raw foods are known to have higher concentrations of omega-3 and omega-6 fats, such as purslane and walnuts.

Polyunsaturated fats are the most fluid and least stable of the fats. They have a lower melting point and are susceptible to oxidation and rancidity. The essential fatty acids omega-3 and omega-6 are both polyunsaturated. The need for omega-3 and omega-6 fatty acids is well established and highly promoted these days. There is an ideal balance between omega-3 and omega-6 that is supportive to health. The ideal ratio for intake is around 1 to 2, omega-3 to omega-6.

There are some variations in the recommendation, but studies have proven that the more unbalanced omega-6 you have in your diet compared to omega-3, the more inflammation occurs and the higher the incidence of coronary heart disease. Omega-3 fatty acid consumption is severely lacking in most American diets, and the consumption of grains and grain-fed animals is the major cause. As a result, most people consume 10 to 20 times more omega-6 than omega-3. Removing grain-fed meats and grain-based foods from your diet is a major step toward achieving a better balance. Chia seeds, flax seeds, spinach, and blue-green algae are foods that have more omega-3 than omega-6. Other foods that have a healthy balance of both fats are hemp seeds, pumpkin seeds, walnuts, and zucchini.

Monounsaturated fats are characterized by one double-bonded molecule (one unsaturated bond) in the fatty acid chain while all the other bonds are single-bonded. They can be categorized between the very stable saturated fats and the unstable polyunsaturated fats. Monounsaturated fats are more stable and less susceptible to rancidity than their polyunsaturated kin. Monounsaturated fats remain liquid at room temperature and become solid in the refrigerator due to their higher melting point. Olive and sesame oil are good examples of monounsaturated fat. Foods that provide a high amount of healthy monounsaturated fats are olives, avocados, sunflower seeds, sesame seeds, and macadamia nuts.

Dangerous Saturated Fats

Saturated fats are given their name because they have no double bonds, and the fatty acid chain is completely saturated with hydrogen atoms. People are familiar with saturated fats because of their consumption of dairy products and flesh foods. These animal-based sources of saturated fats remain solid at room temperature. Cheeses and bacon fat are common examples. Animal-derived saturated fats contain cholesterol, and plant-derived fats contain none; however, saturated fats are heat tolerant, making them a better choice for cooking. Heating oils, no matter how stable, produces harmful byproducts. Clearly, on a raw food detoxification program, we are happily avoiding this danger.

Micro-Nutrients

While macro-nutrients are known as carbohydrates, proteins, and fats, the smaller nutrients that make up these larger nutrients are called micro-nutrients. Many organic micro-nutrients are common vitamins and minerals. This category of nutrients is further divided into macro-minerals and micro/trace minerals.

Unfortunately, cooking, heating, and processing turn many life-sustaining, organic compounds in raw foods into useless, inorganic compounds. Foods that are fortified with vitamins and minerals are typically fortified with unusable inorganic compounds, which is why it's important to eat a variety of nutrient-dense, chemical-free raw foods. As a source for both macro- and micro-nutrients, raw food can't be beat.

Micro- and Macro-Minerals

Although most people are familiar with different types of vitamins, minerals often get much less attention and are worth getting to know a bit better. The distinction between micro- and macro-minerals is determined by the daily amount required for health. Most of the macro-nutrients are consumed in quantities greater than 100 micrograms a day. The big four macro-minerals are present in all organic (living) compounds and are consumed by default as we eat, drink, live, and breathe:

- Oxygen

- Nitrogen

- Carbon

- Hydrogen

All the other organic life-giving minerals are bound to the big four. In isolation, minerals such as calcium are plant food, but when bound to the big four through absorption and utilization by plants, they become organic people food. The organic macro-minerals that we get from raw foods are as follows:

- Calcium

- Chloride

- Magnesium

- Potassium

- Phosphorous

- Sodium

- Sulfur

Raw foods are loaded with these minerals in different concentrations. All green, leafy vegetables contain high amounts of calcium while garlic and onion have high concentrations of sulfur. Adjusting your intake of raw foods to meet deficiencies can be as easy as modifying your diet to include more of a nutrient-dense food until a healthy balance is achieved. Eating more dark leafy greens will quickly raise your intake of calcium, for example.

Micro-nutrients are required in amounts less than 100 micrograms a day: cobalt, copper, iodine, iron, manganese, molybdenum, nickel, selenium, and zinc. These trace elements are critical for health. For example, a deficiency in iron results in anemia while a deficiency in iodine results in goiter. Both of these conditions are completely preventable by eating a variety of raw foods. Iron-rich foods are leafy greens (especially spinach) while iodine-rich foods are the sea vegetables.

> **FRESH FACT**
>
> Some unusual trace minerals in the human body include arsenic (As), vanadium (V), nickel (Ni), cobalt (Co,) and tin (Sn). Although arsenic is most commonly known as a poison, in trace amounts it is part of our natural biology and poses no threat.

Coloring Our Lives

"Antioxidants" is quite a buzzword in the world of health and nutrition these days. What's all the fuss about? An antioxidant prevents oxidation (rust and decay). Oxidation is part of the life cycle in both the organic and inorganic world. The job of antioxidants in our diet is to keep this process in check.

Oxidation from free radicals has a tendency to get out of control if not monitored and managed, and it's the job of antioxidants to manage this process. Antioxidants are most easily identified when we think of our food in terms of color. For example, chlorophyll is the green in greens, beta-carotene is the orange in carrots, and lycopene is the red color in watermelon and tomatoes. The antioxidants in vibrantly colored fruits and vegetables often are concentrated in the skin. This is why it is important to consume chemical-free produce—so you can safely eat the skin. Washing the skin is really not adequate enough to remove these chemicals.

Antioxidants overlap into other nutrient categories, such as enzymes, vitamins, flavonoids, carotenoids, and more. It can be a bit confusing, but realize that raw foods naturally contain antioxidants and—as we'll find out when we discuss superfoods in Chapter 17—some extremely high concentrations of these beneficial antioxidants.

There are two major classifications of antioxidants related to how we assimilate them:

- Water-soluble antioxidants
- Fat-soluble antioxidants

Water-soluble antioxidants in excess are excreted from the body while fat-soluble antioxidants can be stored for later use. Antioxidants, whether fat- or water-soluble, have been shown to alleviate, stop, and even reverse symptoms associated with aging as well as many chronic conditions. The positive press regarding antioxidants has been and continues to be newsworthy, but the antioxidant-rich foods that are part of your raw food detox program are simple foods that have proven themselves over the centuries.

Antioxidants and Their Food Sources

Antioxidants	Food Sources
Water-Soluble	
Vitamin C	Citrus, camu camu, rosehips, greens, mangoes
Catechins	Green tea, raw chocolate, grapes, raisins
Glutathione	Apples, asparagus, avocadoes, broccoli, carrots, garlic
Punicalagins	Pomegranates
Anthocyanins	Açai berry
Resveratrol	Grape skins, mulberries, peanuts
Xanthones	Mangosteen
Fat-Soluble	
Vitamin E	Almonds, corn, cold-pressed oils, dulse, greens
Vitamin A (carotenoids)	Apricots, carrots
Lycopene	Tomatoes, pink grapefruit, watermelon
Lutein	Apples, apricot, beets, corn, kale, peach, spirulina
Zeaxanthin	Corn, goji berries, grapes, spirulina, zucchini
Beta carotene	Apricots, broccoli, goji berries, mango, nori, papaya, tomato

Fiber

Fiber is one of the nutrients we consume that is exclusive to plant life (there is no fiber in flesh foods). We are consistently told that we can never get enough of this marvelous substance. What exactly is fiber, and how can it help us get and stay healthy?

Types and Purpose

Fiber comes in two types: soluble fiber and insoluble fiber. Fruits and vegetables contain a variety of soluble fiber while grains contain insoluble fiber. Soluble fiber is an essential nutrient that the body cannot create on its own, and it's critical for optimizing nutrient absorption and elimination. Soluble fiber is a bulking agent, which absorbs water and expands within the digestive tract. This serves two important purposes: moving digested food efficiently through the digestive tract, and binding sugars to enable them to be released slowly in the intestines, which helps prevent blood sugar spikes (associated with diabetes).

Pectin, guar, and mucilage are three types of soluble fiber. Pectin can be found in many fruits while guar is found in the seeds of the following plants: guar, carob, fenugreek, and tara. Most people are familiar with guar gum, which is used as a thickener in ice cream and other products.

Mucilage is found coating chia, flax, and psyllium seeds. Just add water to a teaspoon of seeds to see this soluble fiber in action. The soluble plant fibers in mucilage are unique in that they can relieve constipation and can also relieve diarrhea. Both chia and flax are used as foods while psyllium is considered a fiber supplement not known for anything other than its high concentration of mucilage.

Insoluble fiber is best characterized by the hull that surrounds grains (such as wheat) and oats (known as bran). Bran contains a portion of the nutrient profile in whole grains, especially oils, which makes bran and whole grains subject to becoming rancid. This was one of the primary motivations for refining grains, which separates the bran and leaves a more stable, less-nutritious product. Insoluble fiber is unaffected by water and passes through the digestive system intact. Bran tends to be abrasive and irritating to the digestive tract and can be troublesome for those who have health conditions such as colitis or other gastrointestinal conditions caused by bowel irritation. Processed cereals and bran supplements have unnaturally high concentrations of harsh and abrasive insoluble fiber and can potentially be implicated in a number of digestive dysfunctions.

I often hear from individuals who have digestive disturbances that they "don't do well with raw fruits and vegetables." The blame is often placed on the uncooked fiber in raw foods. In many instances, the efficiency with which raw foods cleanse the body is often confused with being an irritant. Raw food author Paul Nison was able to heal himself of Irritable Bowel Syndrome (IBS) with the raw foods that his conventional doctors had warned him he would never be able to eat.

Where to Find It

Soluble and insoluble fiber isn't difficult to find when eating raw foods. Raw, plant-based foods are whole foods, which contain both forms of fiber. Some foods contain more of one than the other, so it's important to eat a variety of whole foods. Enjoy the soothing benefits of soluble fiber in fruits such as plums, prunes, peaches, okra, and mangoes; in vegetables such as celery, kale, and spinach; and in seeds such as chia and flax. Many fruits, vegetables, nuts, and seeds contain a good amount of insoluble fiber, which passes through the digestive tract intact.

The Least You Need to Know

- The raw food detoxification program will easily meet your nutritional needs.
- A variety of the macro-nutrients—carbohydrates, proteins, and fats—can be found in the edible plant world, providing you adequate protein and calories while eating a plant-based diet.
- Micro-nutrients, including vitamins and minerals, and antioxidants, which can help maintain vibrancy and health, are plentiful in raw foods.
- Fiber, an essential nutrient, is found in both soluble and insoluble forms in a raw food diet and can be obtained only from the plant kingdom (unlike other nutrients).

Healing Foods and Superfoods

Chapter

17

In This Chapter

- Choosing local and wild produce
- The wonders of sprouts and wheatgrass
- Super-powerful superfoods

Eating well and eating raw will be valuable to your health in many ways, but getting to know the power of healing foods and superfoods can really make a difference in your future vitality and toxin-free life. From eating local produce to learning about more unusual foods you can add to your diet, this chapter will help you explore the possibilities.

Foods That Heal

By now, you are well aware of the healing power of raw foods. Some of the most powerful healing foods, however, grow vigorously in the wild—often in extreme conditions—and many of them have yet to be cultivated. These hearty plants stand out from the rest of the plant world because they make do with less and are usually referred to as "weeds" by most of us. But many can actually be consumed safely if you know what you are picking. Plants such as purslane and dandelion greens actually hold powerful nutrition in their weedlike appearances.

Making the effort to learn about and harvest wild edibles can be a rewarding experience. In our modern times, not everyone can learn botany and traverse jungles to harvest wild foods. There is a practical solution, though. A class of foods is readily available that contains some of the same exotic and wild properties, and you'll be able to find it in your healing food search at local health-food stores, grocers, and farms.

Organic Considerations

Ideally, for raw food detoxification to be successful, you need to eat raw foods that are toxin-free, which means choosing only organically grown foods.

Statistics collected from the USDA Pesticide Data Program and the FDA Pesticide Monitoring Database show data regarding toxic chemical residue on conventionally grown produce. Another alarming statistic shows that fruits and vegetables were often contaminated with multiple chemical toxins. In a particular review, some samples of celery, strawberries, and blueberries tested positive for traces of 13 different chemical toxins! While each toxin may be present in trace amounts (less than one part per million), also consider the synergistic effect of combining toxins.

> **DETOXER'S ALERT**
>
> Toxicological synergy refers to the combined effects of multiple toxins. Although safe levels are set for some single chemicals, when combined their toxicity can potentially be magnified dramatically. Pesticides and herbicides are tested individually to compile minimal safe exposure levels. This "safety number" is not realistic, however, because in the real world, the use of only single toxins in chemical farming is rare. In almost all cases, multiple chemicals are sprayed on plants and soil.

Clearly, organic produce is the way to go whenever possible. But there is also another rule of thumb you could incorporate into your buying habits that will help remedy any toxic concerns—and is often fresher, packed with more nutrients, and potentially less expensive. Start to get to know the advantages of staying local.

Local Farming

"Locavore" is a recently invented term to describe someone who consumes locally produced goods. Buying locally has multiple benefits for the consumer, retailer, and ultimately the planet. Raw foods should be consumed at their absolute peak of ripeness, when they contain the most flavor and nutrition. Vital nutrients and the life force within living foods begin to decrease once the food has been picked from the plant. The longer it takes for the food to go from the farm or tree to your mouth, the less vitality the food has.

Local foods contain specific nutrients that are part of the local landscape as well. The local characteristics are supportive to the consumers' health in that region. When transporting foods across the planet, many fruits are actually harvested in an unripe state and allowed to ripen in transit to the grocery store. This works out fine for the food distributor, but it's not ideal for the consumer.

Depending on where you live, there are various options for buying local produce. After decades of obscurity, the farmer's market has reappeared as an excellent opportunity to buy locally. By purchasing from local growers, you know you're getting produce that is fresh and have the opportunity to ask questions regarding their farming practices.

RAWESOME TIP

Once you've found a local market and food growers you trust, you might even be able to go one step further. Many local farmers will actually allow you to visit their farms and see where all the magic happens.

Purchasing from local vendors also helps stimulate the local economy. There has been a trend in recent years of large, multinational corporations buying smaller farms. This corporate takeover of family farms has brought an end to family traditions that have spanned generations. The farmer's market has been a blessing to those remaining family farms that have hung in there over the years. Many of these farms are part of the historical and cultural fabric of their local communities, and their continued existence depends on community support.

Where the Wild Foods Grow

There is something special about collecting wild-growing foods. Wild foods contain a vigor that farm-raised foods just don't have. Wild harvesting or foraging are terms used to describe the collection of edible plants from the wild. This may be a park, a wooded lot, or even your yard.

Common and delicious wild greens are dandelion, nettle, purslane, sorrel, malva, clover, and plantain. Many herbs grow wild, such as garlic, rosemary, mint, and fennel. Other tasty edibles are the more obvious fruits, such as blackberries, raspberries, blueberries, grapes, figs, loquats, and mulberries. Wild foraging is a fun way to reconnect with the natural foods that grow abundantly around you. Studies of the nutrient content of wild foods show them to be dramatically more nutritious than their domesticated cousins.

Adhere to some basic, commonsense principles when wild harvesting, however. Know for sure that what you are harvesting is edible! There are numerous stories of people harvesting foods, particularly mushrooms, in their own areas without being aware of the toxicity—so always consult with a local expert. Also, know that what you are picking hasn't been sprayed with chemicals. Just because it appears to be in the wild doesn't mean someone hasn't been treating the area.

Farmer's markets and some local grocery stores may carry wild edibles. Care should be taken, though, to identify wild edibles. Keep in mind that just because they aren't poisonous doesn't mean they are worth eating. Also, you may come across foods labeled "wild-crafted" as you explore the world of raw foods. You must be aware that this term has no regulation or standardization behind it. Wild-crafted foods are collected from the wild, yet there is no guarantee that they are chemical free or superior to organically grown foods. Take caution with your purchases and talk with other locavores to discover the best sources.

The Best of the Bunch

With so many raw foods to choose from, how do you know which ones will work best for you? Selecting the best foods for your personal raw food detox plan can start with utilizing the chemical-free whole foods available to you in your area. Here are some suggestions.

Top Ten Whole Foods

Depending on where you live, your supply of organic produce or access to farmer's markets may be limited. This shouldn't deter you from undertaking a raw food detox, though. Many supermarkets will carry produce and items upon request. It's worth asking to see whether your local store is willing to supply some healthy alternatives. Here's a quick list of some of the most common fresh, organic, and farmer's market produce you can easily find and use in your detoxification program:

Apples	Kale
Berries	Melons
Celery	Onions
Citrus	Spinach
Cucumber	Sprouts

Honorable Herb Mentions

When thinking of produce, don't forget about herbs, which can be powerfully healing and contain numerous healthful properties and nutrients. They are another easy way to ramp up the healing potential of your raw food detox. Many herbs can be grown indoors on window sills or outside in containers. Herbs can not only add spice to your cuisine but also a splash of green to your home environment. Here's a list of some of the easiest herbs to add to your detoxification program:

Basil	Mint
Cilantro	Parsley
Garlic	Turmeric
Ginger	

Sprouts: Big Nutrition, Small Package

Eating sprouts is a great way to take advantage of the storehouse of nutrition locked away inside nuts, seeds, and legumes. In their dried and dormant states, these foods keep a portion of their nutrition hidden. Sprouting releases this nutrition and activates the powerful enzymes they contain.

Sprouts have been recognized as an ideal food source since before 3000 B.C.E. They are a complete protein source and contain a full spectrum of nutrients. Sprouts are a biogenic food, which means they are capable of creating life. Biogenic foods are one step up from bioactive foods, which are the enzyme-rich raw and living foods that are part of the raw food detox program.

 FRESH FACT

During the ocean travels of Captain James Cook, sprouts were brought along to prevent and remedy scurvy because of their high content of vitamin C. Sprouting was the ideal proposed solution developed to alleviate protein shortages in the United States during World War II. The food shortages never occurred, and the plan was never enacted.

To follow the raw food detox program, you won't need to learn sprouting—although it can be easily done at home (or even in your car!). We focus more on incorporating sprouts into your meals, whether they are piled on top of salads, stuffed in a sandwich, floating in your soup, or tucked away inside wraps. Sprouts are available in most grocery stores and include varieties such as sunflower-seed sprouts, lentils, mung bean, broccoli, alfalfa, clover, and more. Some sprouts are spicy while others are milder.

Ann Wigmore

Often referred to as the "Mother of Living Food," Ann Wigmore (1909–1994) was a holistic health practitioner, nutritionist, author, and living foods advocate. She believed in the power of raw and living foods for health, healing, and longevity, and sprouts and wheatgrass juice were at the heart of her healing practice. She co-founded the Hippocrates Health Institute with Viktoras Kulvinskas in 1968, and today there are several healing centers around the world that follow her health teachings:

- Ann Wigmore Natural Health Institute, Puerto Rico

- Ann Wigmore Foundation, San Fidel, New Mexico

- Hippocrates Health Institute, West Palm Beach, Florida, and Mayacamas, California

- Creative Health Institute, Michigan

- Living Foods Institute, Atlanta, Georgia

- Living Foods Wellness Center, Michigan

- Optimum Health Institute, San Diego, California, and Austin, Texas

- Mitzpe Alummot, Israel

- Tree of Life Rejuvenation Center, Patagonia, Arizona

Wheatgrass

Wheatgrass and wheatgrass juice is something you may have seen at a health-food store or juice bar. Essentially sprouted wheat grown in soil or hydroponically (in water) and harvested and juiced while it is still a young grass, wheatgrass is nothing short of phenomenal. It has the same chemical makeup as human red blood cells (hemoglobin) except that blood contains iron, which makes it red; wheatgrass contains magnesium, which makes it green.

Wheatgrass juice is a complete protein loaded with minerals and enzymes and revered for its potent healing properties. Chlorophyll is responsible for part of the magic of wheatgrass. This green plant pigment aids in red blood cell production, detoxification, boosting the immune system, and alkalizing the body. The list of the reported benefits from consuming wheatgrass is long and impressive:

- Improved digestion
- Elimination of body odor
- Anti-viral
- Anti-fungal
- Balancing blood sugar
- Reversal of aging signs
- Improved dental conditions
- Improved vision
- Reduced inflammation
- Alleviation of depression

Kulvinskas praises wheatgrass in his book *Survival into the 21st Century:* "In therapeutic amounts, it will detoxify the body by increasing the elimination of hardened mucous, crystallized acids, and solidified, decaying fecal matter. Wheatgrass juice's high enzyme content helps dissolve tumors. It is the fastest, surest way to eliminate internal waste and provide an optimum nutritional environment. Wheatgrass juice can also be used as a poultice, wash, douche, or bath, stimulating healthy new cells and fighting infections."

Wheatgrass and its juice can definitely be a matter of taste for many, but if you have the opportunity to try this marvelous healing food, you may be quickly persuaded to add it to your detoxification program and your overall future health regimen.

Home Sprouting

For those of you who would like to explore home sprouting, I recommend sprouting mung beans, buckwheat groats, quinoa, lentils, alfalfa, or clover. This will save you money and allow you to participate in growing your own food. The simplest forms of sprouting can be done on paper towels and in jars. Once you have successfully raised your first crop of sprouts, you may be hooked on sprouting. Sprouting is a great way to reconnect with your food. There are sprouting resources available online and in many books. *The Sprouting Book* by Ann Wigmore is a great place to start, and The Sprout People at sproutpeople.org is also a great resource for sprouting information and supplies.

Super Foods

Some foods have an extraordinarily high concentration of specific vitamins, minerals, or nutrients. These foods stand out from the crowd and are heroes among foods: "superfoods." Some are from exotic places while others are as common as aloe vera, garlic, and miso. It's definitely worth getting to know the entire team and finding ways to incorporate them into your diet.

Crazes and clever marketing have already brought some of these superfoods to the public's attention, along with a large influx of products. Sort through the hype and the natural, bona-fide products in order to gain maximum benefit.

Meet the Team

Açai berries, noni fruit, goji berries, mangosteen, and cacao are some of the items you may see featured and promoted in health-food stores, and they are all superfoods. Even in their processed forms, they can deliver a powerful nutritional boost for a population starved of nutrition. By doing a bit of research and seeking out quality, unadulterated sources of superfoods, you can ramp up your raw detox and rejuvenation potential.

One of my favorite ways to consume superfoods is by blending them into smoothies. It's best to get fresh or dry superfoods in their purest forms (as opposed to powders that feature a blend of different ingredients). There are some superfood blends that are top quality, though. Look for consumer reports and those recommended by natural health-care practitioners. Avoid cheap supermarket brands that are loaded with unpronounceable ingredients and chemical fillers.

Here are some of the greatest superfoods available:

Açai	Garlic
Aloe vera	Ginger
Bee pollen	Goji berries
Blue-green algae	Maca
Cacao	Miso—unpasteurized
Camu camu	Noni
Chia seeds	Royal jelly
Chlorella	Sea vegetables
Fermented foods—unpasteurized, such as sauerkraut and pickles	Spirulina

Superfoods and Raw Food Detox

So how do superfoods fit into the raw food detox equation? They're the glue that holds the new you together. Superfoods are there to fill in the cracks and to make sure all your nutritional bases are covered (with room to spare). If optimizing your nutrition is like throwing darts, then using superfoods is like throwing a dart that is twice the size of the dartboard, from two feet away. It's not cheating; it just ensures that you'll always win.

In the introduction to David Wolfe's book *Superfoods*, he writes, "Eating superfoods is a way to guarantee that you will get the nutrients you require to be healthy all the years of your life. Because superfoods are natural, they provide an abundance of synergistic elements in their natural state that work together in the human body in ways that scientists have not yet begun to fully comprehend."

Try to get to know as many of these wonderful allies as you can. You'll be super glad you did.

The Least You Need to Know

- Healing foods and superfoods can be terrific allies in your quest for optimal health during and after your detox program.

- Getting to know your local farm produce as well as wild produce with the help of a local expert will help not only your detoxification efforts but the local farmers and community as well.

- Sprouts and wheatgrass have been touted as essential to good health.

- Superfoods such as açai and goji berries can make a remarkable difference in your health efforts and should be added to your diet whenever possible.

Living Foods

In This Chapter

- The benefits of fermented live foods
- Prebiotics and probiotics examined
- Great sources for supplementing your diet

A powerful class of foods, known as living foods, contributes a surplus of life to the body. These foods are highly valuable to good health and can easily be incorporated into your diet. You've probably already heard a bit about them—substances such as fermented foods, probiotics, and prebiotics. Getting to know these plant-based foods will help you get the most from your raw food detoxification program.

In this chapter, we explore living foods in detail and learn why they can be a vital part of restoring health and keeping you detoxified. From fermentation to cultures to healthy bacteria and the food that feeds them, you'll learn about this life-giving force.

Fermented Foods and Cultures

Fermentation is the name given to the controlled or uncontrolled process in which microorganisms (bacteria and fungi) break down complex substances into smaller units while also creating new substances. This process of bacterial transformation is going on everywhere in the natural world. You may not see it, you may possibly smell it, but it's happening. The medium to be consumed (food) and environmental conditions determine who shows up to the fermentation feast. Microbes have their specialties, meaning that controlling the food source and environmental conditions can dramatically effect which microbes come to roost.

The first living foods were discovered by accident, and although the mechanism for the living nature of these first ferments was unknown at the time, people realized there was something special about them. We now know and have studied the workings of fermentation and living foods, which are an invaluable food-processing and preservation method. A distinction needs to be made, however, between living ferments and dead ferments.

> **FRESH FACT**
>
> Early alcohol fermentation was probably discovered by accident when grapes or grain were left in the sun and bacteria in the air landed and began the process of making wine or beer.

The Living and the Dead

Commmon foods that employ fermentation in their production are: yogurt, cheese, bread, alcoholic beverages, tofu, miso, soy sauce, tamari, sauerkraut, kimchi, vinegar, and kombucha. The healthy microbes in foods are referred to as probiotics, which we'll look at in greater detail later in the chapter. Of the foods mentioned previously, however, almost all are consumed "dead." This is because pasteurization turns dairy ferments into dead foods while baking kills the yeast in breads. Fermented bean and vegetable products such as sauerkraut, kimchi, tofu, and miso are often heated to kill the microbes employed in fermentation— thus extending shelf life. But microbes are an integral part of all life (yours included). The quantity, quality, and ratio of microbes in and on our bodies as well as in the environment determine the health of a system, so completely destroying them—as is the case in most dead fermentations— is not what we want.

Fortunately, a fermentation renaissance has come about in recent years. Creative impulses, quality concerns, and health benefits all are motivating factors for fermenting at home. By doing so, consumers of living fermented foods can take advantage of the health benefits. Health-food stores and even large supermarkets are beginning to carry unpasteurized fermented foods due to demand from the consumer as the value of living foods and ferments is understood.

Microbe Allies

Microbes are an integral part of our lives and our health. Actually, it has been shown that excessively sterile conditions can be detrimental to health. Part of the reason is because microbial, and particularly natural microbial, balance plays an important role in immunity. Children and adults who are deficient in the proper balance and amount of internal microbes suffer numerous health challenges, including digestive troubles and lowered immunity. Having a trillion-strong team of healthy bacteria working symbiotically with you is a huge health aid. Our bacterial companions protect us by competing with pathogenic organisms and also by conditioning our immune systems. Cultivate and populate your inner terrain with a wide variety of bacterial cultures by consuming living foods.

DETOXER'S ALERT

Some fermented foods contain a very high amount of *Lactobacillus* bacteria, which produce lactic and acetic acid as byproducts. For many, these acids can produce an overly acidic condition in the body, so fermented foods such as kimchi, sauerkraut, and kombucha should be consumed in moderation.

Probiotics

Probiotics are the healthy bacteria that inhabit our digestive systems (specifically, the colon). They are critical for proper digestion, the assimilation of nutrients, immunity, nerve function in the intestine, and a host of other important health processes. Probiotics have been shown to be effective in remedying all types of digestive issues, including diarrhea, Irritable Bowel Syndrome (IBS), allergies, asthma, dermatitis, and indigestion. Unpasteurized living foods that have been created by the process of fermentation are full of healthful probiotics.

Friendly Flora

Our bodies are host to more than a trillion microbes—the highest concentration of which live inside our large intestines. These probiotics, also known as internal flora, work with us symbiotically—not unlike the microbes that live in the soil. Soil-borne microbes condition the ground, feeding on decaying material and inorganic minerals to create an ideal environment for plants to grow. Both plants and soil microbes benefit from this arrangement because the microbes feed on inorganic compounds and decaying matter (dead plants and animals), which feeds the plants. The plants eventually die, feeding another generation of microbes who feed the next generation of plants.

Something quite similar to this process occurs inside our body every day. In the soil, the proper balance of microbes in nutrients provides support for the growth of plants, which utilize and concentrate the soil's nutrients—binding them with carbon molecules and transforming them from inorganic compounds into organic compounds, which we are then able to consume. Once we consume these plants, the soil/microbe scenario gets turned outside-in. These natural foods are assimilated into the body through the process of digestion, of which the probiotics in our digestive tract are an integral part. Our internal environment and the partially digested food nourish the microbes in our digestive tracts, and the microbes return the favor by breaking down compounds, supporting immune function, and fending off unhealthy pathogens.

Antibiotic Activity

Antibiotics are the destroyer of microbes, which can be a good thing. Unfortunately, they don't discriminate in the destruction of both harmful and beneficial bacteria. Although antibiotics can be life-saving in the case of severe infection, they can also cause a host of problems.

The overuse and abuse of antibiotics has resulted in drug-resistant strains of microbes that can actually wipe out a person's internal flora. In the case of overuse of antibiotics, the microbes left behind are typically harmful. These microbes that were once an oppressed minority now have the opportunity to expand their influence and wreak havoc in the body. Candidiasis, generally described as a yeast infection, can result from antibiotic-caused imbalances. Microbial competition is the only thing that keeps the internal balance in a healthy system and opportunistic pathogens such as Candida in check. The best way to guard against unwelcome bacterial infection is to nurture a healthy inner terrain and eat a good variety of living foods that contain healthy bacteria.

Once you've prepared your inner terrain for healthy probiotic inhabitation through a raw food detox, it's then time to invite them into their new home. Eating predominantly alkalizing, chemical-free raw foods will help get things started and encourage healthy flora to thrive. A sure way to get the good guys in and push the bad guys out is by eating cultured foods and by taking probiotic supplements.

Prebiotics

Prebiotics are the foods that support the growth of probiotics. After a detox, you'll want to create a welcoming environment for probiotics to flourish. Prebiotics are similar to putting out a birdhouse and birdbath and planting flowers to attract birds. This makes the new terrain inviting for habitation.

Food for Flora

Prebiotics are most commonly a form of plant fiber. A food is not called a prebiotic, but it may contain prebiotics and consequently be a good source. The two main prebiotics you may hear about are oligofructose and inulin. Being that prebiotics are newly discovered, there is still some debate in classifying them—but it is widely agreed that something that increases the number and activity of internal bacteria can be designated a prebiotic. As a rule, prebiotic sources are almost always from raw sources—and none are animal derived.

FRESH FACT

Prebiotics were discovered and named by Marcel Roberfroid in 1995. He defined them as "a selectively fermented ingredient that allows specific changes, both in the composition and/or activity in the gastrointestinal microflora that confers benefits upon host well-being and health."

Vital Benefits

Because our health depends on the healthy balance of our internal terrain, it would make sense that substances such as prebiotics that support probiotics would benefit overall health. Studies already show that prebiotics play a vital role in digestive and overall health. Results have shown that prebiotics have a positive effect on calcium and other mineral absorption, immune system support, internal pH support, the reduction of colorectal cancer, balancing regularity, and the alleviation of Crohn's disease and ulcerative colitis. Prebiotics make happy flora, happy flora makes a happy gut, and a happy gut makes a happy and healthy you.

Here are the top 10 sources of prebiotics. The percentages listed show how much of each source is made up of prebiotics.

- Raw chicory root: 64 percent

- Agave powder: more than 50 percent

- Yacon powder: more than 50 percent

- Raw Jerusalem artichokes: 31 percent

- Raw dandelion greens: 24 percent

- Raw garlic: 17 percent

- Raw leeks: 11 percent

- Raw onions: 8 percent

- Cooked onions: 5 percent

- Raw asparagus: 5 percent

Sources of Living Foods

Sauerkraut, kimchi, miso, apple cider vinegar, and kombucha are the easiest living ferments to obtain from a health-food market or grocery store. All of these are relatively easy to make at home for those of you who are ambitious. All of these living foods need to be refrigerated to inhibit further fermentation, however. Due to the preserving nature of fermentation, living foods can be stored for months and even years at proper temperatures. Here are some of the best-known living foods you can add to your diet.

Sauerkraut

Sauerkraut is fermented cabbage prepared in Eastern European, particularly German, tradition. Sauerkraut can be as simple as pickled green cabbage or as elaborate as a combination of root vegetables; garlic; onion; and spices such as caraway seeds, juniper berries, and celery seeds. The variations for making sauerkraut, as with all fermented vegetables, are endless. The procedure for making friendly ferments such as sauerkraut and kimchi naturally fortify them with an array of nutrients and a high concentration of Lactobacillus bacteria. Fermented cabbage has been shown to have higher-than-normal concentrations of *isothiocynates*, which are known to fight cancer.

FRESH FACT

Captain Cook brought sauerkraut on his voyages because its high vitamin C content prevented scurvy among his sailors. Limes were the choice of the British navy while the German navy used sauerkraut. Hence, British sailors were referred to as "limeys" and German sailors as "krauts."

Kimchi

Kimchi is the Korean equivalent to European pickled/fermented cabbage. Historians have traced the practice of fermenting cabbage back to China, so kimchi most likely has been around longer than sauerkraut. Regardless of its origin, kimchi is usually spicy and hot because of its copious amounts of garlic, ginger, and hot peppers. Studies have shown that kimchi has powerful immune-boosting properties.

Miso

Miso is a fermented bean paste that most people are familiar with in the form of miso soup. Too often, the soup—made with boiling water—is dead, so watch the temperature to gain the benefit. Heating water and miso to no more than 120 degrees Fahrenheit and allowing it to cool will make soup that is warm and alive.

Miso takes indigestible protein sources—beans, legumes, and pulses—and makes them digestible. The bean most commonly used to produce miso is soybean. Because of GMO concerns, you must purchase organic miso products to ensure that you are not consuming a food containing genetically modified ingredients. Chickpea miso has no soy. Be sure to try all different varieties if you can. Miso must be unpasteurized to retain its health benefits, so look for it in the refrigerated section of your health-food store.

Miso contains Lactobacillus, just like the other friendly ferments. This probiotic has been shown to protect against E. Coli, Salmonella, and Shigella. Another beneficial characteristic of unpasteurized miso is its capability to detox heavy metals and radiation from the body. Miso is an enzyme-rich, protein-dominant food containing all the essential amino acids. Miso contains omega-3 fats as well as lecithin (an emulsifier). This combination allows miso to balance cholesterol in the body. Miso is also a great source of calcium and B vitamins. Use as much miso as you can, even after your raw food detox, to maintain vibrancy and health.

Kombucha

Kombucha is a fermented, sweetened tea that employs a colony of bacteria and yeast to consume sugars and transform the tea mixture into a living drink. The microbe colony responsible for this friendly ferment forms a gelatinous layer that floats on the surface of the tea. This floater is referred to as the "mother" of living vinegars and is often referred to as SCOBY, an acronym for "Symbiotic Colony of Bacteria and Yeast."

The result of fermenting kombucha is an acidic tea with a sweet and sour flavor that reminds many of vinegar. During the fermentation process, natural carbonation occurs as well as the production of a small amount of alcohol (usually less than 0.5 percent).

As with all living foods, enzymes, probiotics, and concentrated nutrients engender these foods with health-supporting properties. Research in Russia and Germany has shown kombucha to be supportive of digestive function. Other potential benefits include support of detox organs, immunity support, cancer prevention, and improving liver function. Although many stand behind the reported benefits of kombucha, the medical establishment warns that these claims are as yet unsupported through extensive testing or human trials.

Living Foods and Raw Food Detox

Fermented, living foods combine a multitude of healing factors in a concentrated form. On their own, fermented foods—when added to a cooked-food diet—can aid in digestion and help repopulate the gut with healthy bacteria. With raw food detox, living foods work synergistically with raw foods to ramp up detox, aid digestion, boost the immune system, reestablish healthy flora, and support overall wellness.

Added Benefits

Living foods are just another level of support for detoxification and reestablishing balance in the body. With the list of choices mentioned, one can easily incorporate living foods into the daily diet. Try starting your day like 75 percent of the people in Japan with a warm bowl of miso soup instead of coffee. Enjoy kombucha during the middle of the day as an energizing snack, and add fermented vegetables to your nightly meals.

What to Expect

Some potential side effects can occur when adding living foods to your diet, such as indigestion, gas, or even diarrhea. As discussed previously, these are all common cleansing reactions that occur when the body expels toxins and brings itself back into balance. Observe how your body responds to these foods, and modify your intake to a comfortable level.

All the fermented foods mentioned are concentrated in flavor and effectiveness. Fermented vegetables are often too sour/acidic to consume in excess, miso is too salty to be eaten without thinning with other ingredients, and a bottle of store-bought kombucha is labeled as containing at least two or more servings. Fermented foods are whole foods, but their concentrated flavor and healing potential should be taken into consideration when portioning servings.

The Least You Need to Know

- Living foods, which are the result of fermentation and cultures, are vital to good health.
- Friendly bacteria and flora present in the digestive tract help maintain gastro-intestinal regularity and immunity.
- Prebiotics and probiotics can be obtained from living foods such as sauerkraut and miso and should be included in your diet even after detoxification.
- Experiment with the addition of living foods to your eating program to see how your body reacts and to explore different methods of preparation to get the most from their flavor and benefits.

The Newly Detoxed You

Now that you've completed your program, you'll want to maintain your success—and in this part, you'll find out how. From continuing to eat a percentage of raw food or actually becoming a raw foodist for life, you'll get the scoop on how to do it. There will also be plenty of information about seasonal flushes and cleanses that you may wish to try, and finally you'll learn about ways to keep your home environment toxin-free as much as possible with healthy types of fabrics, gadgets, and additions to your surroundings.

Seasonal Cleaning

In This Chapter

- All about juice fasting
- Enhancing your detox experience
- Popular cleanses and flushes

Building lasting health takes time and effort. Once you've detoxed your body and created a healthy new you, some seasonal practices can help you maintain radiant health. This maintenance can be done periodically or even during your raw food detoxification.

Juice fasting can be a great relief for the digestive system, while other types of flushes and cleanses are directed at specific organs in the body and the removal of certain types of toxins. Let's take a look at some methods for keeping you cleansed and healthy.

Fasting

When most people think of a fast, they assume that it requires complete abstinence from all food and even water. Many religious fasting periods entail at least a period of time in which food is not taken in order to appreciate and focus on specific spiritual practices.

Fasting, however, can also be done simply with juices, and we will discuss this type of fasting in this section.

The vital components of fresh fruits and vegetables are pure water, macro- and micro-nutrients (carbohydrates, fatty acids, proteins, vitamins, minerals, and antioxidants), and fiber (soluble and insoluble). Although fiber serves an important role in transporting food nutrients through the intestines and provides something for the musculature of the intestines to work against, it is not something we want the body to cope with during a fast. Juicing separates the fiber from the water and nutrients in the item being juiced so that the body is relieved of the burden of having to extract the nutrients from the fiber during the digestive process.

All About Juicing

Fruit and vegetable juicing enables a person to take in more hydration and nutrients than he or she would normally consume if eating all the items in un-juiced form. All the nutrients present in juices are absorbed in the stomach and small intestine, so there is no need for the juice to pass into the large intestine because there are no solids or insoluble fiber to eliminate. This translates as "vacation time" for many of the body's systems. The stomach is relieved of the burden of secreting hydrochloric acid and other digestive enzymes, and the pancreas gets an enzyme break as well. Fruit and vegetable juices contain only small amounts of fat, which are broken down by the food enzymes contained in the juices. This means the liver can take a break from its digestive duties.

What do all these vacationing organs do during their time off? They clean house, of course. "Vacation time" in the body equates to detox and revitalization time. Juicing provides the ultimate opportunity for this process to occur. But know that juicing works properly only if you're consuming fresh, unprocessed juices such as the ones in Chapter 15 and not pre-made, pasteurized fruit and vegetable juices.

 RAWESOME TIP

You don't need to fast to enjoy freshly prepared juices. They can be consumed prior to meals, as a snack, or as a meal replacement. Having a juice in place of dinner is an effective way to maximize your body's ability to detox and repair itself at night.

Feast Versus Famine

Fasting on freshly prepared juices has been referred to in recent years as juice feasting—especially when done at home while continuing your daily and weekly schedule. Juice feasting puts no limits on the amount of fresh juice one can drink during the course of a day. This is especially useful if you need to continue your daily and weekly tasks while juicing. A person can still get the benefits of hydration, mineralization, and optimization of weight while juice feasting. Detoxification of the body will also occur with juice feasting—but on a less-dramatic scale than if you were to follow a strict detoxification program.

While enjoying a juice feast, a person will still experience fluctuations in energy levels and mild cleansing reactions. Although an individual may continue his or her weekly tasks, he or she should take great care to respect the signals the body is sending. It's best to back off the intensity and amount of tasks done in a day when juice feasting to accommodate cleansing and detox. The ideal way to experience juice fasting is to set time aside completely devoted to juicing and healing.

Juice fasting is best done when you can completely unplug from the duties of daily life. Often, people go to a healing spa or retreat center to engage in a fast and cleanse. Under these conditions, everything is prepared and all you have to do is adhere to the daily schedule. This is the ultimate way to say "I love you" to your body. Many of the guests at cleansing spas report that throughout the year, they remain immune to seasonal illnesses.

Not everyone can hop a plane and fast for a week, though. That is where raw food detox comes in. It brings together a number of health-supportive practices, which you can adopt into your daily life wherever you are. Each of these practices on their own is extremely powerful, but it's when they're combined that healing happens on an exponential scale.

Water Fasting

Raw food detox does not recommend water fasting. Water fasting is an advanced form of healing that can do more damage than good if an individual is not properly prepared for the experience. The high level of stored toxins in the bodies of most people, combined with a low level of vital nutrients, creates a dangerous combination when considering a water fast. Water fasting deprives the body of vital nutrients, thus causing the body to enter a catabolic state in which complex compounds are broken down into simpler forms so they can be consumed as energy. In the case of water fasting, these complex compounds are muscle tissue, fat, and even bone. When deprived of external nutrients, the body will cannibalize itself to maintain its vital functioning. If a person is already nutritionally in the hole, then water fasting can lead to life-threatening deficiencies. Juice fasting and feasting, on the other hand, are safe and effective ways to provide nutrients, hydration, and detoxification.

DETOXER'S ALERT

Water fasting should only be considered with proper supervision and guidance from a healthcare professional.

Cleansing Programs

Eating a diet of predominantly raw foods is an effective cleansing program, especially if it's high in whole foods such as fruits and vegetables. The hydration, nutrient, and fiber content of plant foods aids the body in returning to a healthy balance. There are also cleansing programs, however, that can be used independently or in conjunction with the raw food detox diet. Herbal cleansing programs come in a variety of forms that are customized to your level of commitment. Some can be done while eating your regular diet while others require a modified diet or fasting. The Master Cleanser, also known as The Lemonade Fast, is a simple DIY cleanse that has been around since 1976 and has been used by tens of thousands of people to heal many chronic conditions. Also, there are mono-diet cleanses that focus on eating one fresh, healing food for a specific duration.

This brief overview of the variety of cleanses is meant to pique your interest and introduce you to some of the cleansing possibilities. To do your body justice and honor your health, investigate the pros and cons of any cleansing program and come to your own conclusion while also consulting a specialist in the field.

The Herbal Cleanse

A seven-day fasting and herbal cleanse program known as Arise and Shine was created by Richard Anderson ND, NMD after publishing the books *Cleanse and Purify Thyself Books One and Two*. My personal experience with this herbal cleanse was so positive that I returned six months later and did it again, although this time I had been eating a diet of at least 60 percent raw foods. My results were even more positive, which proved that I was doing something right. This herbal cleanse, along with many others, is available online and at health-food stores.

An herbal cleanse is usually a kit that contains a variety of cleansing mixtures (powders, liquids, and capsules) that are to be taken in stages over a period of three to five weeks. Over the course of the program, you can expect to strengthen digestion and cleanse the organs of the body, including the colon, liver, gall bladder, and kidneys. These cleanses focus on eliminating "unwanted guests," which are the buzzwords for bacteria, mold, yeast, fungus, and parasites. Herbal formulas usually consist of a variety of herbs and natural ingredients known for neutralizing and eliminating these substances.

The Master Cleanser

The Master Cleanser, also known as The Lemonade Diet, may be the easiest way to become introduced to the health benefits of fasting. This program, documented in the early 1970s by Stanley Burroughs, involves only a few simple ingredients and a set of directions that anyone can follow. Lemons, grade-B maple syrup, and cayenne are at the core of The Master Cleanser.

The Master Cleanser Procedure

10 oz. spring or purified water—warm

2 TB. lemon or lime juice (fresh squeezed—not bottled)

$\frac{1}{10}$ tsp. cayenne pepper, or to taste

Maple syrup to taste

1. Mix water, lemon or lime juice, cayenne pepper, and maple syrup in a glass.

2. Make a large batch for your daily needs. Drink 6 to 12 glasses a day.

3. Pure water, as well as peppermint tea, may be consumed between lemon drinks.

4. Drink an organic laxative tea at bedtime.

5. Drink a Salt-Water Flush first thing in the morning. (Directions follow later in the section.)

The designer of The Master Cleanser does not recommend the use of enemas or colonics. His intestinal cleansing method of choice is the Salt-Water Flush. The most important ingredient for this internal salt bath is the salt. Do *not* use iodized table salt; it is not supportive of health when consumed with food or for flushing the digestive system. Use chemical-free sea salt that has been sun dried or Himalayan pink salt for the flush and all other salt needs. If iodine deficiency is a concern, consume kelp or dulse flakes and other sea vegetables to meet your iodine needs.

The procedure for the Salt-Water Flush is as follows:

1. Dissolve 2 teaspoons healthful salt in 1 quart warm purified water.

2. Drink entire quart first thing in the morning on an empty stomach.

3. The salt and water mixture should pass through your system in about one hour. Be prepared for several eliminations.

4. Adjust the amount of salt (more or less) if necessary to achieve a mild flushing of the intestines.

This simple method for flushing out the digestive system is safe, cheap, and effective. The combination of the lemonade mixture throughout the day, laxative herbal tea before bed, and salt-water flush each morning enables the body to perform a deep cleaning that can easily be done from 10 to 40 days. The fresh lemon juice provides much-needed minerals, especially sodium, while also dissolving mucus in the body. Lemon juice is very alkalizing as well and helps restore the acid/alkaline balance in the body. The maple syrup provides calories for energy in the form of simple sugars. Grade-B maple syrup also provides important minerals for the body. Cayenne pepper adds a potent kick to The Master Cleanser by breaking up mucus and dilating blood vessels, which aids in cleansing and the elimination of toxins. The simplicity and effectiveness of The Master Cleanser has made it the most popular of all the different cleansing programs.

As an aside, some other notable cleansing and fasting practices worth mentioning are herbal parasite cleanses, mono-meal fasting, and The Purifying Diet. If you are curious about any other fasting and cleansing programs, be sure to investigate them thoroughly before embarking on any new plan and always consult with a physician.

The Least You Need to Know

- Seasonal cleaning, consisting of juice fasting and certain types of cleanses, can be an adjunct to a successful detoxification.

- By resting the digestive tract and its need to cope with plant fiber, juicing gives your body a chance to recoup its vitality and perform detoxification on its own.

- Cleanses from herbal to the popular lemonade flush may be desirable as a supplement to your detox program.

- Any type of fasting or cleansing should be embarked upon with caution and the approval of a health professional.

Maintaining Your Success

In This Chapter

- Keeping up your newfound health
- Eating raw is a long-term option
- An introduction to advanced raw food prep techniques

If you've reached this far and have successfully completed your detoxification program, you should definitely pat yourself on the back. You may be wondering, however, what to do now.

In this chapter, we look at ways you can easily maintain your success by eating a certain percentage of raw foods and avoiding pitfalls that might set you back. In addition, for those who are considering a lifetime of raw food eating, there are some tips and advanced techniques.

I Did It! Now What?

The duration and depth to which you take your raw food detox experience is up to you. At the beginning of the program, it is important to have clear health goals in mind. You can modify these goals along the way. Eventually, you will reach a point where you'll step back and assess the results. If you like what you see, you'll want to know how to maintain what you have created. Just like cleaning out the garage or a messy closet, once it's cleaned out and organized, it has to stay that way. Without maintenance programs, things fall into disrepair—and you end up back where you started.

Staying in Place

Keep in mind that improvements can always be made now that the major work has been done. But staying in place is the most important thing to work on. Hopefully, many of the raw food menu items and ingredients were enjoyable enough for you to adopt into your everyday life. There are also the daily and weekly exercise activities that you may have already embarked upon. The bottom line is that if, after the raw food detox program, you end up keeping any new eating or exercise habits, you'll most likely be able to maintain your success. You'll be able to notice the difference in how you feel when you eat something heavily processed. These little hints will encourage you to maintain the new level of health you worked patiently to achieve.

Avoiding Backsliding

Holidays and family events can pose a challenge for anyone trying to diet—never mind maintain a healthy raw food diet. Once you've finished the program, these family events are likely to be a challenge still. Be sure that you are prepared with an ample supply of strategies and foods, as discussed in Chapter 8. If you like, give some of the old family standards a try again in small amounts, see how your stomach reacts, and determine whether you want to incorporate them periodically into your new way of eating.

Backsliding is sometimes only temporary and occurs during special events or emotional issues, so don't despair. Be aware of how you are treating yourself, the emotions you are experiencing, and other circumstances that may be involved. Now that you know how raw food detox, cleansing, and fasting work, you are prepared to handle almost any instance of backsliding. It's not about falling down, it's about getting back up. You've done a great service to your personal health and well-being. Keep up the good work.

The 60-Percent Solution

If you've made it through the raw food detoxification program, you've experienced numerous days of eating 100 percent raw. Looking back, how challenging was it? If you think it was easy or only mildly challenging, then maintaining a diet of 60 percent raw foods will be a piece of cake (raw cake, of course!)

The 60-percent solution is even easier than the Program A menu. If you're capable of doing a higher percentage of raw foods, then go for it. If you eat one meal a day raw and the rest of your meals with a raw component, you're likely to be close to 60 percent. Don't worry so much about the numbers; just be aware of how you feel. If you make a point to eat at least 60 percent raw and 100 percent whole foods, you'll not only maintain your health but likely continue improving it.

Light Steaming and Cooking

When you re-enter the world of cooked food, remember what you learned about the detriments and toxins created by certain cooking methods. You should be well aware of the things to avoid. If you need a refresher, then just remember to stay clear of high-heat grilled, microwaved, and fried foods. Your best options for cooking are steaming; baking; or stir-frying (with a wok) using a combination of water, tamari, and high-heat oils. Remember to enjoy the raw portion of your meal before eating the cooked stuff, and be extra mindful of food combining—especially when eating cooked foods. Continue to eat a good variety of nutrient-rich fruits and vegetables that are colorful and diverse.

Going All the Way

It is entirely possible that when you come out on the other side of your raw food detox experience, you just might want to continue doing raw foods at 80 percent to 100 percent. Congratulations! Eating a highly raw diet is a practical and effective way to maintain and continue your personal health transformation.

Diet Advice for Raw Food Newbies

Matt Monarch refers to a 100 percent or highly raw diet in his book *Raw Success* as a lifetime fast. That doesn't mean you'll be starving yourself; rather, you will be constantly cleansing your body's systems. Everyone has toxins to remove from their systems, and how toxic your life was prior to the raw food detox program will determine what amount of cleansing you will experience along the way. It's a matter of listening to your body and making dietary adjustments according to these signals.

Hopefully you've taken the opportunity during the raw food detox program to explore other information available regarding the raw food diet and lifestyle. *The Complete Idiot's Guide to Eating Raw* is a great place to find valuable information and more than 150 raw recipes for continued raw eating. Be sure to look at the resources in the back of this book and explore online resources as well.

Advanced Raw Food Prep and Eating

If you want to experience raw foods on a deeper level, try some of these more
advanced raw food preparation practices. As part of a long-term raw food diet, they
are indispensable and add a tremendous amount of variety and taste to your new way
of eating:

- **Sprouting:** Sprouting is an easy way to incorporate more raw foods into your
daily life while actively participating in the growing process. Sprouts are easy
to grow and packed with biogenic life-force energy. Some of the simplest
sprouts you can grow are sunflower seeds, buckwheat, quinoa, mung beans,
and lentils. To sprout seeds and beans, you need to soak them first. The type
of seed or bean determines the amount of time they need to be soaked. Nuts
can be soaked and germinated, but they won't actually sprout. Soaking nuts
and seeds increases the bioavailability of their nutrients.

- **Fermenting:** Fermenting foods such as nut or seed cheezes and even vegetables such as kimchi and sauerkraut is an advanced but fun practice. There
are also a variety of fermented drinks, such as kombucha, kefir, and Rejuvalac.
Check out Sandor Ellix Katz's book *Wild Fermentation* for detailed information, instructions, and fermentation recipes.

- **Dehydrating:** Dehydrated foods often take the place of those crispy and
baked snacks we used to love so much. It can get expensive buying raw
crackers, granola, and snack bars. Once you try kale chips, you're going to
be hooked. Most people who take a liking to raw foods eventually invest in
a dehydrator. This low-heat "hot box" enables you to make a variety of raw
recipes that couldn't be made any other way. In some cases, the dehydrator
enables you to dry salads and fruits that would otherwise spoil. By drying
these foods, you can make preserved snacks that last for weeks and even
months.

Falling Back and Trying Again

If at first you don't succeed, peel a mango and try again. Raw food detoxers who
become raw food enthusiasts have chosen an adventure that isn't always predictable.
It's not uncommon to have some setbacks or to visit old foods just to see how they

treat you. Keep learning, experimenting, and experiencing the joy of raw foods. Don't be afraid to ask for advice from other raw foodists or health specialists. There's a support network of people who are experiencing a journey similar to yours. In many cases, when you look for advice, you may find yourself able to *offer* advice as well.

How Often Is Safe?

If you find yourself constantly struggling with food issues and the self-discipline of staying raw, then there may be some deeper issues you need to work through. It's normal to move forward and plateau or move forward, stop, and then slide back a little before moving forward again. Your dietary choice becomes an issue only if mental and/or physical harm is experienced. People often ask, "How often is it safe to come off and on the diet?" That depends on the individual as well as his or her current health challenges and goals. Be sure to consult with a professional if you find yourself having difficulty sticking with the program for whatever reason. Avoid extremes. If you have chosen one direction and you decide to change directions, do it gradually and listen to the feedback your body provides.

Getting It Right This Time

There's no secret to getting a raw food lifestyle right. If "right" entails feeling good physically and emotionally while radiating health, then getting it right means doing whatever it takes to achieve this goal. Healthy, sustainable foods are only one aspect. Yes, food matters—but it isn't the only part of the equation. If you find yourself in a continual pattern of highs and lows, then there is likely some aspect of your life that needs attention and adjustment. It could be physical, mental, emotional, or a combination of all three.

Some people find that fasting on delicious green juices and fruit-juice blends helps them get more motivated and on track than simply eating a limited percentage of raw food. You can always do a single-day juice fast and streamline your diet. The Program D menu is a liquid fast that can bring you a certain level of clarity and balance and may be the best way to jump-start yourself and get it right this time.

The Least You Need to Know

- After your raw food detoxification, maintain your newfound health and vitality with regular checks on your eating habits and lifestyle.

- Eating a 60-percent raw food diet can be enough to maintain your success, incorporating simple and light cooking techniques.

- If you decide to embrace a totally raw eating regimen, you can learn an enormous amount from fellow raw foodists and other resources.

- A slip or back-step in your program can be easily remedied by getting back on board with healthy raw meals and juice fasting.

- Those hoping to be long-term raw food enthusiasts should explore the techniques of sprouting, fermenting, and dehydrating to enhance their eating pleasures and experiences.

Detoxing Your Life

In This Chapter

- Keeping the new you healthy and detoxed
- Learning about natural clothing fibers
- Creating a toxin-free home

Toxins may be a fact of life, but that doesn't mean you are powerless against them. So far, the raw food detoxification program has helped you address toxins in your food and water. Now it's time to deal with those external toxins that are often less apparent but just as big of a concern as the ones you can ingest.

Identifying potential toxic influences can help you prevent future health problems. Both an ounce of wheatgrass and an ounce of prevention can go far toward protecting you from everyday toxins.

The New You

Now that you have successfully addressed the inner environment of the body, let's look at some of the external changes you can make to support your hard work. There are a number of environmental toxins that you can avoid and eliminate. Let's take a tour around the house and see what positive changes you can make that will be easy and result in less toxic stress on the new you.

Natural Fiber Clothing

The clothing you wear is your second skin, and while your first skin is your largest organ and a key player in the detoxification process, it would seem counter-productive to adorn it in fibers that are anything less than natural. Cotton, linen, hemp, and silk are some of the natural fibers available in clothing, but be aware that they should also be chemical free. Here's a quick look at some of the fiber options you should consider:

- Cotton

- Linen

- Hemp

- Bamboo

According to the Organic Consumers Association latest fact sheet, cotton is the most toxic crop on the planet, using 25 percent of the world's insecticides and 15 percent of the world's herbicides! This is a startling statistic, considering across-the-globe cotton represents only 3 percent of all farming. In the United States, 75 percent of the cotton grown is genetically modified. As we touched on earlier, GMO crops have been shown to be dangerous not only as a food source but also to the environment. These facts alone should make you think twice before buying anything but organic cotton. Although it is natural, unless it is also chemical free and organically grown, it could result in toxic exposure and stress on your body.

Made from linseeds, which are commonly known as flaxseed, linen is a good choice for the natural fiber wearer. Although more expensive to produce than cotton, linen boasts two to three times cotton's strength and has a cooling effect when worn (which is why it is a popular summer clothing fiber). Linen tends to wrinkle quite easily, but it's still worth considering. Its primarily toxic-free, organic production, unless colored with unnatural dyes, makes it a highly desirable fabric.

Hemp is a very durable and functional fiber produced from the plant of the *Cannabis* genus. (Hemp is not to be confused with marijuana, which is grown specifically for its psychoactive properties.) As a material, hemp has become more and more popular because of its numerous advantages. It has even been acknowledged as a type of miracle crop because of its rapid growth, high yield, resistance to pests, capability to recondition the soil, and the all-around usefulness of all parts of the plant. Although the United States is the world's biggest importer of hemp food, beauty, and clothing products, it has yet to lift restrictions on the farming of hemp due to its unfortunate connection with marijuana.

Bamboo is not only a sustainable building material but is also being turned into sustainable fabrics. In the past, bamboo production techniques were cost prohibitive, resulting in an expensive end product. With the development of new production methods, bamboo fiber clothing is now a planet- and people-friendly reality. Bamboo is actually a type of fast-growing grass. Because of its hardy nature, it can easily be grown organically. Some of the appealing qualities of organic bamboo clothing are its wicking (water absorbency) capability and its tendency not to cause allergic reactions to those sensitive to other plant fibers. It also boasts strength and antibacterial properties. All of these characteristics combine to make bamboo fiber ideal for being worn next to the skin.

Energetic Accessories

What you carry around as an accessory is as important as what you wear on your body when it comes to toxic exposure. Most of us keep our cell phones, iPods, laptops, and numerous other items practically glued to our persons. But the potential for electromagnetic field (EMF) toxicity could be significant.

The potential health effects of the very low-frequency EMFs surrounding power lines and electrical devices are the subject of ongoing research and public debate. In workplace environments, where EMF exposures can be up to 10,000 times greater than the average, the U.S. National Institute for Occupational Safety and Health (NIOSH) has issued some cautionary advisories but stresses that the data is currently too limited to draw good conclusions. Other nongovernmental-connected factions have suggested that EMFs can contribute to everything from cancer to Alzheimer's.

What can you do to protect yourself from this possible hazard? Numerous devices are available that call themselves EMF protection devices. They come in almost every shape, size, and color and are made from both natural and manmade materials. Some plug into your wall, and others you wear around your neck. Do these EMF protection gadgets work? Much of the "science" behind these devices is questionable, although many of the products come with a full technical explanation of how they work and testimonials to support efficacy claims. Investing in a personal EMF protection device is partially a leap of faith. Plates, double-terminated quartz crystals, and a recently devised Quantum Balance Crystal are some of the remedies being touted these days to protect you. For most of us, simply becoming less addicted to all things high-tech could prove helpful.

Your New Environment

If your home is your castle and your body is a temple, then we all have a good deal of real estate to maintain! The raw food detox program should have you up to speed on how to manage the health of your body with whole-food nutrition, cleansing, and detox. The home environment can be maintained in a similar way as well. There are a variety of simple additions and modifications for the home to create a health-supportive environment.

Himalayan Salt Lamps

Glowing pink Himalayan salt lamps have grown in popularity in recent years. Not only do they add stylish soft-light illumination, but they also give off negative ions. The light bulb inside the salt lamp heats the pink salt, causing it to give off negative ions that bind with airborne toxins and remove them from the air. Negative ions aren't unique to salt lamps—they're found in nature as well. They are present in forests, at waterfalls, and where there are crashing waves on the oceanfront. It's interesting to note the appeal of these natural outdoor settings. Maybe it's the negative ions that are partly responsible for the allure and appeal.

Houseplants

The benefit of having living plants in your home environment is highly understated. Salt lamps can add illumination and give off negative ions, but plants provide a brightness of their own while filtering the air. Studies have shown that the addition of plants to a room improves the mood and lowers the stress level of the occupants. Houseplants also exchange carbon dioxide for oxygen and filter all the air in your home while removing toxins such as benzene, formaldehyde, and trichloroethylene. Their ability to filter indoor air is so potent that NASA researched hundreds of plants to find which ones are most effective at cleaning the air. Their conclusions were: English ivy, spider plant, peace lily, golden pothos, snake plant, Chinese evergreen, weeping fig, heartleaf philodendron, elephant ear philodendron, and the rubber plant.

Air Filtration

If houseplants are too high maintenance for you, you may want to look into getting an air-filtration system for your home. Filters are available that can clean the air of a single room or even an entire house. Some are capable of ionizing the air, and others use zeolite, HEPA filters, carbon, electricity, and/or ultraviolet (UV) light to eliminate airborne toxins. Price, capacity, and method of cleaning vary between different filtering units.

Water Filtration

The toxins that are potentially spilling out of your tap water can have a dramatic impact upon your health. Clean water is not only important for drinking and preparing foods but also for bathing. Your skin is your largest organ of elimination, but it also has the ability to absorb substances it comes in contact with.

Distilled water is one of the safest options for consumption. Reverse osmosis (RO) filtration is another good choice. With RO systems, maintenance is required to assure the system is working properly. There are also a variety of other water-cleaning options using technology similar to air filtration. Some of these systems eliminate certain toxins while not affecting others. Countertop units that filter water only in the kitchen are available. Cheap spigot-attached filters are useful but less effective than countertop units.

In the bathroom, a shower filter is the easiest option for protecting yourself from potential contaminants in your household water. If you can afford a whole-house filtration system, then you are covered in both the kitchen and the bathroom. Shop around and try different types of systems before selecting one. While affordability is a major consideration, taste is another aspect to consider—so be sure the final product is something you will be happy drinking.

You're Grounded!

Many of us heard this saying when we were children, and we always thought of it as a bad thing—but in reality, being *grounded* is good for us. The benefits of being grounded come back to the negative ion factor and health. Health, in its most basic form, is a balance of all the forces that act upon us, both seen and unseen. Negative ions are the balancing force that offsets positive ions, which cause oxidative stress, free-radical damage, and aging. Grounding takes advantage of the fact that the earth is a grounding source of negative ions, while radiation from the sun and EMFs represent a source of positive ions. When you are connected to the ground, these opposite forces are neutralized and balanced. You literally discharge built-up positive ions when you become grounded, and it is a feeling that is actually noticeable. Studies have shown the efficacy of grounding on normalizing blood pressure and heart rate and alleviating inflammation.

The simplest method for grounding oneself is to walk barefoot outdoors, preferably on grass, sand, or dirt. Grounding can occur on manmade surfaces, but you should avoid direct contact with some surfaces such as asphalt, which is petroleum based. Swimming in the ocean, lakes, and streams grounds you; even showering will ground you if the pipes used in the plumbing are metal. Last, being in contact with trees and bushes that have roots extending into the ground will ground you. So yes, hugging a tree does have therapeutic benefits!

Unfortunately, many of us live insulated lives and are rarely grounded at all during the course of the day. Potentially, the only time many of us get a good grounding is when we take a shower. Think about how energized you feel after a shower. Part of that feeling is likely caused by being freshly grounded.

Aside from walking barefoot in nature, swimming outdoors, and hugging trees, you can use grounding technologies in your home. One of these items is a grounding mat, which you can place your bare feet on while you are at home or at work. The mat plugs into the wall's electrical socket and takes advantage of the ground (third-prong) portion of properly installed electrical wiring. The grounding mat enables you to remain grounded even at the top of a skyscraper office building. Author and health advocate David Wolfe says he travels with his grounding mat in his carry-on luggage, and once he gets off a plane, he plugs it into the first outlet he can find and grounds himself.

Another similar grounding technology is simply a grounding bed sheet. Made from cotton with silver fibers sewn into it, the sheet has wire that attaches to it that enables you to connect to the grounding socket on a standard wall outlet. The effect of the grounding sheet is like sleeping on the bare ground. One company that makes these products is called Barefoot Connections.

Staying Inspired

There are many speakers, authors, and raw food chefs who were and continue to be a motivational force in my life and may provide similar inspiration for you. I found early encouragement to make personal life changes and raw food choices by reading books by the Boutenkos (*Raw Family*, *Eating Without Heating*, and *Greens for Life*), David Wolfe (*Sunfood Diet Success System*), and Gabriel Cousens (*Rainbow Green Live Food Cuisine*). I've continued to expose myself to inspiring influences not only in the world of health and nutrition but in the areas of green living, spirituality, and personal growth.

If you immerse yourself in these inspirational works and become motivated to continue your path of healthy living, you may even wind up being an inspiration to someone else.

In the end, it comes down to finding your passion. It's funny how things evolve in one's life when you are able to find your passion and choose a path that supports personal growth. Completing the raw food detox program may be the boost you need to start you on that new path of self-discovery.

The Least You Need to Know

- You can continue the detoxification process and keep on a healthy path by exploring ways to detox yourself on the outside.
- Choosing natural fibers to wear and avoiding as much electromagnetic field activity in your immediate environment as possible will help to keep toxins at bay.
- Salt lamps, house plants, and air- and water-filtration systems are all good ideas for keeping your home environment toxin free.
- Stay inspired by reading and exploring more ways to get healthy, and continue the great work you have already accomplished.

Glossary

acidosis   the opposite of alkalosis, a condition where there is excessive acid in the body solutions.

acrylamide   toxin produced in food as a result of various cooking processes.

acupuncture   ancient healing practice using needles inserted at specific points on the body to restore balance and move energy.

acutonics   a form of acupuncture using sound and tuning forks to move energy in the body.

adaptive secretion of enzymes   biological law stating that the body will change the amount of digestive enzymes produced according to the requirements of the food consumed.

adaptogens   natural substances that balance the systems of the body.

advanced glycation end products (AGEs)   toxic byproducts created by some methods of cooking.

aerobic   requiring oxygen.

aerobic exercise   exercise that increases the rate of respiration and circulation for a sustained period of time.

alkalosis   the opposite of acidosis, a condition where body fluids become overly alkaline.

amino acids   building blocks of protein.

amylase   a starch-splitting enzyme.

anabolic process   the process of building up organs and tissues, which occurs in living organisms.

anaerobic   not requiring oxygen.

anandamide   also known as the "bliss chemical," a cannabinoid found in raw chocolate.

ancestral eating   also known as the Paleo Diet and Cave Man Diet, a form of eating that focuses on uncultivated, unprocessed, and natural foods.

anemia   an illness associated with an iron deficiency.

anti-inflammatory   a compound that reduces inflammation in the body.

antibiotics   natural or synthetic compounds that kill microbes and are often used to fight bacterial infection.

antioxidant   a compound that prevents free-radical damage and oxidation.

Antoine Béchamp   French biologist who supported the theory that internal environment dictates health or wellness, not the invasion of external germs.

aromatic isothiocyanate   a compound found in foods such as maca that has been shown to have aphrodisiac properties.

assimilation   the incorporation or conversion of nutrients through digestion.

Ayurvedic   an ancient Indian health practice; the Sanskrit term means "the science of life."

bentonite   a clay derived from volcanic ash that has both industrial and therapeutic uses for absorbing toxins.

Bifidobacterium   a variety of friendly bacteria that exists symbiotically in the human body; one of the strains found in human breast milk.

bioactive   having an effect on a living organism.

bioavailable   the degree and rate at which a substance is absorbed into a living system or is made available at the site of physiological activity.

biogenic   resulting from life or living things.

biophoton the ultra-weak light emission from living organisms.

bran a type of insoluble fiber surrounding grains.

bromelain a protein-splitting enzyme found in pineapple.

buffer the use of alkaline minerals to neutralize acids in the body.

Candida a genus of yeast that is present in the human body.

candidiasis (candidosis, thrush) a yeast infection caused by *Candida albicans.*

cardiovascular exercise Also known as "cardio," this type of workout raises the heart rate.

catabolism process in which larger molecules are broken down into smaller units to be utilized by the body as energy.

Cave Man Diet see *ancestral eating.*

cellulose insoluble fiber that makes up the cell wall of plants.

centenarian an individual living to or past the age of 100.

centrifuge juicer a juicer with a spinning basket.

certified organic term referring to a farming practice that meets established organic requirements.

cheeze word used to describe non-dairy, raw, vegan cheese made with nuts and/or seeds.

chelation a process that helps draw out heavy metal toxins from the body.

chlorophyll the green pigment in plant life that is responsible for photosynthesis.

cleanse a healing practice that focuses on the cleaning of a specific organ or body system.

cleansing reaction physical response by the body to the removal of toxins; common reactions are headache, runny nose, fever, and lethargy. Reactions subside once toxins are removed.

coffee enema   potent method of cleansing the colon and liver by injecting a coffee solution into the colon.

colema   a large-volume enema (colonic), which uses a simple gravity-fed system to deliver water to all parts of the colon.

colema board   board specifically designed for administering a colema.

colitis   inflammation of the large intestine.

colon cleanse   general description for practices that focus on cleaning out the colon, often involving enemas or colonics.

colon hydrotherapy   a healing practice where water is introduced into the colon for the purpose of removing potentially harmful decaying matter.

colon irrigation   see *colon hydrotherapy*.

colonic   see *colon hydrotherapy*.

degenerative disease   a disease characterized by progressive changes in tissue.

denature   to modify the molecular structure of a substance through chemical or physical processes.

detox reaction   see *cleansing reaction*.

detox symptom   symptoms and reactions that may occur while toxins are being eliminated from the body.

detoxification   also called detox; the removal of toxins from the body.

diseases of civilization   diseases associated with manmade toxins, unnatural living, over-consumption, and over-indulgence.

diverticula   small balloon pockets that are unnaturally formed in the bowel.

diverticulitis   infection that occurs in diverticula.

dry fast   a fast during which one abstains from both solid food and all liquids, including water.

earthing   a term created that refers to ground technology and connecting to the earth's resonant frequency.

electrolyte liquids containing conductive minerals that are necessary for proper health and hydration.

electromagnetic field (EMF) an energy field created by electrically charged objects that has the potential to harm living organisms.

elimination removal of waste solids and liquids from the body.

empty calories junk foods that contain little to no nutritional value yet are a source of calories.

emulsifier chemical compound that emulsifies fats, which enables them to combine with other liquids.

enema insertion of liquid into the rectum.

enzyme inhibitor molecules that bind to enzymes and decrease or halt their activity.

enzymes heat-sensitive proteins produced in living organisms that are responsible for initiating vital processes, such as digestion and immune response.

Essene Diet a raw food vegetarian diet practiced by the Essenes and highlighted in *The Essene Gospel of Peace.*

essential amino acids amino acids that the body cannot manufacture: isoleucine, leucine, lysine, methionine, phenylalanine, threonine, tryptophan, and valine.

essential fatty acids (EFAs) natural fats and oils (omega-3 and omega-6) that are not produced in the body and must be taken in through diet.

excitotoxin a toxic compound (neurotoxin) that affects specific receptor sites in the brain.

far infrared (FIR) sauna a sauna that utilizes both infrared and far infrared light to detox the body.

fast to abstain from a particular food or activity for a specific duration.

fat-soluble a substance that requires fat to be dissolved.

fermentation the breakdown of carbohydrates by microbes, which produces a variety of new chemical compounds.

food combining   eating practice that takes into consideration the physiological requirements for digesting different types of foods to allow for ideal digestion and the assimilation of nutrients.

foraging   collecting wild-growing foods

free-radical   highly reactive atom or molecule with an unpaired electron.

friendly ferment   health-sustaining, bioactive, living foods such as sauerkraut, kimchi, and miso.

galactomannon   polysaccharide found in certain plant seeds.

Genetically Modified Organism (GMO)   also known as a genetically engineered organism (GEO), an organism whose genetic material has been altered using genetic-engineering techniques.

germ theory   theory that is prevalent in medicine today and focuses on external "germs" as being the cause for disease.

glycation   process that occurs when a sugar molecule binds with protein or lipid molecules.

glycogen   chains of simple carbohydrates that are present in animals and used as a source of stored energy.

goiter   illness caused by an iodine deficiency.

grounding devices   devices that connect an individual to Earth and its resonant frequency.

healing crisis   a dramatic response in the body to the cleansing of toxins that is longer and more intense than a cleansing reaction.

heterocyclic amines (HCA)   toxic chemical formed from cooking animal protein at high temperatures.

hormone disruptors   any chemical that disrupts or impedes hormone function in the body.

hormones   chemicals secreted by the endocrine system to regulate the function of certain systems and functions in the body.

hygiene hypothesis   theory that not enough exposure to microbes in our natural surroundings can lead to allergies and asthma.

implant   the insertion of a specific liquid into the rectum, typically for health purposes.

inflammation   swelling, heat, and distress that occurs when the body is injured or infected.

inorganic   a chemical compound not derived from a living source and not bound to a carbon molecule.

insoluble fiber   also known as roughage, plant fiber that is not digested by the body.

interleukin   a chemical found in white blood cells that stimulates them to fight infection.

internal flora   the bacteria that live in the human digestive tract.

Irritable Bowel Syndrome (IBS)   disorder that affects the large intestine and results in a number of symptoms, including abdominal pain, bloating, and irregularity.

isothiocyanate   a chemical compound found in cruciferous vegetables that is shown to have strong anti-cancer properties.

juice fast   a liquid fast that features fresh vegetable and fruit juices in restricted amounts.

juice feast   a liquid fast that features fresh vegetable and fruit juices in unrestricted amounts.

juicing   the process of separating vegetable or fruit juice from the fiber inherent to these plants.

kimchi   Korean-style spicy, fermented vegetables.

kombucha   fermented tea.

Lactobacillus acidophilus   probiotic that occurs in humans and many animals.

life force   the spiritual energy present in the natural world and living things.

linoleic   omega-6 fatty acid.

linolenic   omega-3 fatty acid.

lipase   a fat-splitting enzyme.

live/living foods   a term used to describe vegan, raw foods as well as fermented foods, including non-vegan items such as dairy-based kefir, cheese, and yogurt.

living salts   salt that comes from an organic source, such as sea salt or Himalayan rock salt, and has not been heated to extreme temperatures or chemically processed.

locavore   a person who consumes locally produced products and supports local businesses.

lymphocytes   immune system cells.

macro-mineral   minerals necessary for wellness with a daily established need greater than 400 mg.

macro-nutrient   basic components of nutrition: carbohydrates, proteins, and fats, which can be broken down further into smaller components.

Malliard Reaction   the chemical reaction that occurs between an amino acid and a reducing sugar, most commonly seen in the browning that occurs when baking certain foods.

mannose   plant sugar found in aloe vera.

metabolic waste   waste products created by normal cell function.

micro-mineral   also known as trace minerals, nutrition components needed in very small amounts (under 20 mg).

micro-nutrient   nutrients such as trace minerals that are only needed in small amounts.

monosodium glutamate (MSG)   excitotoxin found in many processed foods that has been shown to contribute to a number of neurological illnesses.

monounsaturated fats   fats that are characterized by having one double-bonded molecule in the fatty acid chain while all the other bonds are single-bonded.

mucilage   water-soluble fiber surrounding seeds such as flax, chia, and psyllium.

mucoid plaque   term used to describe layers of encrusted mucus that form in the small and large intestines and harbor pathogenic bacteria, contributing to disease states.

mycelium   the vegetative part of a fungus that is typically underground.

myelin sheath   insulating layer of lipids that surrounds nerves and is present in the brain.

mylk   term used to describe raw, vegan, non-dairy milk made from nuts or seeds.

natural hygiene   a natural-living and lifestyle philosophy focusing on vegan raw food nutrition and abstaining from chemical-based medicine.

negative ions   molecularly charged particles that are present in the air in many natural environments, such as forests, beaches, waterfalls, and after rainstorms.

oil pulling   an Ayurvedic health practice that consists of swishing cold-pressed vegetable oil in the mouth for several minutes.

organic compound   naturally occurring substances that are bound to carbon molecules, typically from a living source.

oxidation   the breakdown of molecules or cells due to the loss of electrons.

Paleolithic Diet   see *ancestral eating*.

peristalsis   muscle contractions in the intestines that move along waste matter.

pH   potential of hydrogen, a measure of acidity or alkalinity based on a scale from 0 to 14.

phase one detox   biotransformation process that occurs to stored toxins in the body, preparing them to be eliminated in phase two detox.

phase two detox   toxins released during phase one detox that are bound to other chemicals to allow them to be eliminated from the body.

phenylethylamin (PEA)   naturally occurring alkaloid found in raw cacao that is known as the "love chemical."

phytonutrients/phytochemicals   naturally occurring substances in plants that play a role in the immunity of a plant; now being acknowledged and studied for their health-sustaining and restoring properties.

polychlorinated biphenyls (PCBs)   a man-made toxin in some food and consumer products.

polysaccharide   a complex carbohydrate.

polyunsaturated fat   fats characterized by having multiple double-bonded molecules in the fatty-acid chain.

probiotic   bacteria supportive of digestive health.

propolis   bonding agent made by bees, which they use to construct their hives.

protease   a protein-splitting enzyme.

ptyalin   a starch-splitting enzyme present in saliva.

pulse   edible seed.

raw foods   uncooked foods, including fruits, vegetables, nuts, seeds, unpasteurized dairy, meats, and fermented foods.

rebounding   low-impact exercise performed by jumping on a mini trampoline.

rejuvenative   substances or actions that have the capability to restore health and youth.

remineralize   the process of reintroducing minerals into the body.

roughage   another word for fiber.

royal jelly   bee product created by the synthesis of honey and pollen.

salt water flush   method for flushing the digestive tract by drinking salt water.

saturated fat   fats that have no double bonds, and the fatty acid chain is completely saturated with hydrogen atoms.

skin brush   natural fiber brush designed for dry stimulation and exfoliating of the skin.

skin brushing a technique that uses a dry skin brush to exfoliate and stimulate the surface of the skin.

soluble fiber plant fiber that forms into a gel when consumed and aids in digestion and elimination.

Standard Affluent Diet (SAD) also known as the Standard American Diet; characterized by denatured and highly processed foods.

stevia an herb used as a low-glycemic sweetener.

superbugs antibiotic-resistant bacteria.

suppository medicinal delivery system inserted into the rectum.

symbiotic a mutually beneficial relationship.

systemic inflammation chronic inflammation in the entire body brought on by injury, toxicity, or infection.

systems of detoxification organs of the body whose primary function is the elimination of toxins.

The Master Cleanser also known as the Lemonade Fast, a liquid fast that consists of drinking fresh lemon juice in water sweetened with maple syrup.

theobromine a bitter-tasting alkaloid found in cacao; similar to caffeine.

toxemia poisoning by bacterial and/or self-generated toxins.

toxicological synergy the combined effect of multiple toxins that often yields an exponentially greater effect than the sum of the effects of the toxins on their own.

toxin any substance that causes damage to a living organism.

trace mineral naturally occurring minerals necessary in small amounts for health.

trans-fatty acids also known as trans fats or hydrogenated fats; a processed fat used in many foods that has been implicated in causing degenerative diseases.

vasodilator a substance that causes the opening and expansion of blood vessels.

water-soluble a substance that can dissolve in water.

wild harvesting   collecting wild-growing foods.

wild-crafted   a label placed on foods that have been harvested from the wild.

zeaxanthin   an antioxidant that is important for eye health and is found in high concentration in many raw foods, such as goji berries, spinach, kale, and corn.

zeolite   microporous, aluminosilicate minerals commonly used as commercial adsorbents; also used as a detox supplement.

Food Combining Chart

The following charts provide guidelines on food digestion times and the types of food combinations that can be beneficial or detrimental to your health.

RAW VEGAN FOOD CATEGORIES AND DIGESTION TIMES

*Note: these are general guidelines based on observed practices that avoid food combinations that ferment in the gastro-intestinal tract and create acidosis and "internal composting" (see *Rainbow Green, Live Food Cuisine* by Gabriel Cousens, MD for an explanation of this concept). There may be some exceptions since not all possible combinations can be represented, but generally these guidelines work to avoid fermentation and acidosis. Some foods have components that fall into more than one category. Sprouting makes a food more easily digested. For example, unsprouted beans digest slower than sprouted, and sprouting converts some of their proteins into carbohydrates. Blended or finely chopped foods digest faster than usual. Unripe fruit digests more slowly. Also, botanically, any produce with a seed inside is considered a fruit, but for food combining purposes some nonsweet fruits such as cucumber are classified as vegetables.

APPROXIMATE DIGESTION TIME	FOOD*
4+ HOURS	**PROTEINS** Nuts, seeds[1], unsprouted peas & beans (legumes), olives, blue-green algae
3 – 4 HOURS	**FATS** Olives; avocados[2]; pressed nut , seed, & plant oils (olive, sunflower, flax, hemp, safflower, coconut, sesame, others)
2 – 3 HOURS	**NON-STARCHY VEGETABLES AND GREENS** Leafy greens (lettuce, watercress, kale, kohlrabi, parsley, chard, cabbage, carrot greens, turnip greens, collards, mustard greens, endive, etc.) , sprouted greens (alfalfa, clover , broccoli , Brussels sprouts, buckwheat, pea greens, sunflower, etc.) , celery, (mildly starchy: beets, turnips, carrots, radishes), broccoli, cauliflower, asparagus, summer squashes, zucchini , sea vegetables, onions, leeks, chives, green beans, artichokes, okra, sweet peppers, eggplant, blue-green algae, etc.
2 – 3 HOURS	**CARBOHYDRATES/STARCHES** Sprouted but not greened grains (buckwheat groats , quinoa, millet, oats, wheat, spelt, rye, etc.), sprouted but not greened legumes (lentils, green peas, adzukis, mung, fenugreek, etc.), SLIGHTLY STARCHY: carrots, Jerusalem artichoke, beans, turnips, parsnips, sweet potatoes, VERY STARCHY: corn, winter squashes, pumpkin, jicama
1-1/2 – 2 HOURS	**ACID FRUIT** Citrus[3], strawberries, pineapple, sour apples, sour plums, cranberries, sour grapes, crab apples, pomegranates
1 – 1-1/2 HOURS	**SUB-ACID FRUIT** Tomatoes, cucumbers[4], apples, pears, peaches, mango, papaya, apricots, cherimoya, fresh figs (not dried), cherries, most berries (blueberries, blackberries, raspberries)
30 – 45 MINUTES	**SWEET FRUIT & SWEETENERS[5]** Bananas, dried fruit (dates, raisins, prunes, figs, apples, etc.) , sweet grapes (Thompson, Muscat, etc.), pears, ripe persimmons, sweet cherries, sweet berries, agave nectar, yacon syrup, raw honey, molasses, etc.
15 – 30 MINUTES	**MELONS, WHEATGRASS JUICE, FRESH SQUEEZED JUICES** Watermelon, honeydew, cantaloupe, casaba, Crenshaw melon, etc. Melons and fresh squeezed juices digest very quickly and should be consumed alone or with water. Avoid sweet fruit juices, although alkalizing and cleansing, the concentrated sugar feeds yeasts, molds, and funguses.

1. Soaking nuts and seeds releases enzyme inhibitors, makes the nuts and seeds more digestible, and is recommended always.
2. Avocados digest in 45 minutes to 2 hours depending on what they are eaten with.
3. Lemons and limes may be combined with foods above them in the chart.
4. Tomatoes and cucumbers are okay to combine with foods above them except for proteins.
5. Sweeteners, even raw vegan, should be avoided, with the exception of Stevia, an herbal sweetener.

RAW VEGAN FOOD COMBINING

Food combining charts can make the concept of eating seem overly complicated, but actually the basic principles are quite easy, and when you understand them it's not a chore to eat proper food combinations. Understand the basic principles first, and then refer to the chart if you have specific questions.

The concept of food combining is this: some foods digest faster than others, and if you eat a food that digests fast with a food that digests slowly, the mixture will ferment, create acidity in the body, and feed harmful parasites, yeasts, molds, and fungi. Eating certain food combinations will neutralize digestive juices, also causing fermentation and putrefaction. Molds and fungi create mycotoxins and produce wastes that feed harmful bacteria and viruses. An acidic internal environment creates a breeding ground for disease in many ways. Nutrients all the way down to the cellular level tend to clump and create blockages in an acid environment, so cells tend to starve and toxins tend to build up, which accelerates degeneration and creates a cascade of unhealthy reactions in the body. By eating a diet high in raw plant material and observing proper food combinations, *acidosis*, as it's called, can be avoided and degeneration can be slowed or reversed.

GOOD COMBINATIONS

> **Proteins & Fats & Leafy Greens & Non-starchy Vegetables & Sprouts & Lemon or Lime**

> **Starchy & Non-starchy Vegetables & Sprouts**

> **Avocado & Greens & Sprouts & Non-starchy Vegetables & Lemon or Lime**

> **Avocado & Sub-Acid Fruit**

> **Acid Fruit & Sub-Acid Fruit**

> **Sub-Acid Fruit & Sweet Fruit**

EAT ALONE

> **Melons, Wheatgrass Juice, Other Juices**

POOR COMBINATIONS

The Worst:

> **Fruit or Sweeteners* & Protein**
> (Fruit or Sweeteners & Nuts, Granolas, Energy Bars, Fruit Smoothies With Nuts/Nut Milk/Protein Powders, Nut Milks & Sweeteners or Fruit, etc.)

> **Fruit or Sweeteners & Sprouted or Unsprouted Grains/Cereals**

Others:

> **Vegetables & Fruit or Sweeteners***

> **Starch & Fruit or Sweeteners***

> **Starch & Protein**

> **Starch & Avocado**

> **Starch & Acid**

> **Acid Fruit & Sweet Fruit**

> **Desserts After Meals**

* Except the herbal sweetener, Stevia

EWG's Shopper's Guide to Pesticides

The information in this appendix was taken directly from the Environmental Working Group's (EWG) Shopper's Guide to Pesticides. You can download a pdf of this list or phone application for free at www.foodnews.org.

Why Should You Care About Pesticides?

The growing consensus among scientists is that small doses of pesticides and other chemicals can cause lasting damage to human health, especially during fetal development and early childhood.

Scientists now know enough about the long-term consequences of ingesting these powerful chemicals to advise that we minimize our consumption of pesticides.

What's the Difference?

EWG research has found that people who eat five fruits and vegetables a day from the Dirty Dozen list consume an average of 10 pesticides a day. Those who eat from the 15 least contaminated conventionally grown fruits and vegetables ingest fewer than two pesticides daily. This guide helps consumers make informed choices to lower their dietary pesticide loads.

Will Washing and Peeling Help?

The data used to create these lists is based on produce tested as it is typically eaten (meaning washed/rinsed and possibly peeled, depending on the type of produce). Rinsing reduces but does not eliminate pesticides. Peeling helps, but valuable nutrients often go down the drain with the skin. The best approach: eat a varied diet, rinse all produce, and buy organic when possible.

How Was This Guide Developed?

EWG analysts have developed this guide based on data from nearly 89,000 tests for pesticide residues in produce conducted between 2000 and 2008 and collected by the U.S. Department of Agriculture and the U.S. Food and Drug Administration. You can find a detailed description of the criteria EWG used to develop these rankings and the complete list of fruits and vegetables tested at www.foodnews.org.

Dirty Dozen—buy these organic:

- Apples
- Bell peppers
- Blueberries
- Celery
- Cherries
- Grapes (imported)

- Kale/collard greens
- Nectarines
- Peaches
- Potatoes
- Spinach
- Strawberries

Clean Fifteen—lowest in pesticides:

- Asparagus
- Avocado
- Cabbage
- Cantaloupe
- Eggplant
- Grapefruit
- Honeydew melon
- Kiwi

- Mangos
- Onions
- Pineapple
- Sweet corn
- Sweet peas
- Sweet potato
- Watermelon

Resources

Further Reading

Keep your mind refreshed and renewed with the help of these terrific books for further reading.

Raw Food Books

Clement, Brian R., and Theresa Foy DiGeronimo. *Living Foods for Optimum Health: Staying Healthy in an Unhealthy World*. Rocklin, CA: Prima Publishing, 1998.

Cousens, Gabriel, M.D. *Rainbow Green Live-Food Cuisine*. Berkeley, CA: North Atlantic Books, 2003.

Graham, Dr. Douglas N. *The 80/10/10 Diet*. Key Largo, FL: FoodnSport Press, 2006.

Jubb, Annie Padden, and David Jubb. *LifeFood Recipe Book: Living on Life Force*. Berkeley, CA: North Atlantic Books, 2003.

Katz, Sandor Ellix. *Wild Fermentation*. White River Junction, VT: Chelsea Green Publishing, 2003.

Mars, Brigitte. *Rawsome*. North Bergen, NJ: Basic Health Publications, 2004.

Monarch, Matt. *Raw Success: The Key to 100% Raw Vegan Longevity*. Granada Hills, CA: Monarch Publishing, 2007.

Reinfeld, Mark, Bo Rinaldi, and Jennifer Murray. *The Complete Idiot's Guide to Eating Raw*. Indianapolis, IN: Alpha, 2008.

Wigmore, Ann. *The Sprouting Book*. New York, NY: Avery, 1986.

Wolfe, David, and Shazzie. *Naked Chocolate*. San Diego, CA: Maul Brothers Publishing, 2005.

Wolfe, David. *The Sunfood Diet Success System*. San Diego, CA: Sunfood Publishing, 2008.

———. *Superfoods*. Berkeley, CA: North Atlantic Books, 2009.

Juicing Books

Calbom, Cherie, and Maureen Keane. *Juicing for Life*. Garden City Park, NY: Avery, 1992.

Meyerowitz, Steve. *Juice Fasting and Detoxification*. Summertown, TN: Book Publishing Company, 1999.

———. *Power Juices, Super Drinks*. New York, NY: Kensington Publishing, 2000.

Murray, Michael T., N.D. *The Complete Book of Juicing*. New York, NY: Three Rivers Press, 1998.

Walker, N. W. D. Sc. *Fresh Vegetable and Fruit Juices: What's Missing in Your Body?* Prescott, AZ: Norwalk Press, 1970.

Cleanse and Detox Books

Anderson, Rich, N.D., N.M.D. *Dramatic Signs of Healing: Cleansing Reactions and the "Healing Crisis."* Medford, OR: Christobe Publishing, 2000.

———. *The Liver: Cleansing and Rejuvenating*. Medford, OR: Christobe Publishing, 1999.

———. *Cleanse and Purify Thyself: Books 1 and 2*. Medford, OR: Christobe Publishing, 1988.

Baroody, Theodore A. Dr. *Alkalize or Die*. Waynesville, NC: Holographic Health Press, 2002.

Burroughs, Stanley. *The Master Cleanser*. Reno, NV: Burroughs Books, 1976.

Howell, Edward, Dr. *Enzyme Nutrition: The Food Enzyme Concept*. Wayne, NJ: Avery, 1985.

Jensen, Bernard, Dr. *Dr. Jensen's Guide to Better Bowel Care.* New York, NY: Avery, 1999.

Meyerowitz, Steve. *Water: The Ultimate Cure.* Summertown, TN: Book Publishing Company, 2000.

Rose, Natalia. *The Raw Food Detox Diet.* New York, NY: Regan Books, 2005.

Walker, Dr. Morton. *Jumping for Health: A Guide to Rebounding Aerobics.* O'Neill, NB: KE Publishing, 2005.

Cookbooks

Levin, James, M.D., and Natalie Cederquist. *A Celebration of Wellness.* San Diego, CA: GLO, 1992.

———. *Vibrant Living.* La Jolla, CA: GLO, 2001.

Useful Websites

Continue to explore the world of raw food and detoxification by visiting these websites.

Health and Nutrition

Natural News
naturalnews.com
Mike Adams provides a wealth of information regarding health and nutrition. This site offers articles, videos, audio, and also an online store with a variety of great products.

Dr. Mercola
www.mercola.com
Dr. Joseph Mercola shares his personal insights on health and wellness.

Self Nutrition Data
nutritiondata.self.com
Do your best to avoid the ads on this Condé Nast website. Self Nutrition Data features some useful tools for analyzing the nutritional makeup of your diet.

Health Renegade Show
renegadehealth.com/blog
Kevin Gianni and Anna Marie Gianni share cutting-edge health information in a fun and enjoyable way.

The Live Food Experience
www.livefoodexperience.com
Adam Graham invites you to join him on his live-food adventures by featuring recipes and information about live foods.

Raw Food Resources and Shopping

United States

Raw Food World
therawfoodworld.com
Raw Food World provides some of the best raw food products available on the Internet. The site is operated by raw foods educator Matt Monarch and is based in California.

Viva Pura
vivapura.net
Viva Pura, located in Arizona, has an assortment of top-quality superfoods and coconut products.

Natural Zing
naturalzing.com
Natural Zing, located in Maryland, is a complete online source for all your raw food needs. They carry foods, supplements, appliances, media, and more.

Raw Guru
www.rawguru.com
Raw Guru, located in Florida, is a one-stop shop for all your raw food needs. It carries foods, supplements, appliances, media, and more.

Ultimate Superfoods
ultimatesuperfoods.com
Ultimate Superfoods, based in California, features a wide variety of top-quality superfoods and Ayurvedic herbs.

Sea Tangle Noodle Co.
kelpnoodles.com
This business, based in California, is the one place for all your kelp noodle needs.

South River Miso Company
www.southrivermiso.com
Offering possibly the best miso in the Western Hemisphere, South River Miso Company ships its miso throughout North America seasonally. The business is located in Pennsylvania.

Canada

Upaya Naturals
www.upayanaturals.com
Upaya Naturals is Canada's largest raw food source and is based in Toronto, Ontario.

Real Raw Food
www.realrawfood.com
Real Raw Food is a Canadian supplier of organic raw foods at wholesale prices. A minimum order is required to take advantage of their low prices. They are located in British Columbia.

Europe

Mamma Earth—UK
mammaearth.com
Mamma Earth is an online store featuring raw foods, supplements, and cleansing and detox products.

Raw Living—UK
www.rawliving.eu
Raw Living features raw foods, supplements, media, equipment, and more. Raw Living was founded by author and raw food promoter Kate Magic.

The Fresh Network—UK
www.fresh-network.com
The Fresh Network is a one-stop shop for all things raw and healthy. The site is affiliated with the publication *Get Fresh!*, which features articles on raw foods, health, and more.

Health XL—Belgium
www.healthxl.eu

Health XL is a Belgium-based Internet shop featuring raw, organic, and natural products.

The Mastercare Shop features an online store providing raw foods, supplements, equipment, consulting, media, and more.

Keimling—Multi-Language Site
www.keimling.eu

Keimling features many different raw and health-related products. The business is based in Germany, and the website is in German, French, and English.

Australia

Raw Pleasure
raw-pleasure.com.au

Raw Pleasure has an extensive online store, community forum, recipes, and more.

Raw Power Australia
www.rawpower.com.au

Raw Power Australia features a wide variety of raw food products. The site was founded by health educators Anand Wells and Runi Burton.

Japan

Life Collection
www.lifecollection.co.jp

If you know how to read Japanese, this is the raw food site for you.

Online Communities

Eighty Percent Raw
eightypercentraw.com

Eighty Percent Raw features a wide array of information and support for people who are interested in healthy eating and living. The site posts new recipes from featured chefs (including myself).

123 Raw

123raw.ning.com

123 Raw is an online community that provides a discussion forum for those who are interested in raw foods and healthy living.

Give It to Me Raw

www.giveittomeraw.com

GI2MR is a community for people who are passionate about harnessing the power of raw foods and holistic living.

Raw Food Society of British Columbia

www.rawbc.org

The Raw Food Society of British Columbia is a non-profit organization whose aim is to provide information, motivation, and support for those who are interested in vegan raw foods. The site features a calendar of events, online resources, and a community forum.

Inspiration

The Best Day Ever

thebestdayever.com

This is David Wolfe's longevity and media blog. The Best Day Ever provides some of the most cutting-edge information available in the world of longevity, health, and wellness.

Success Ultra Now

successultranow.com

Nick Good and Michael Mackintosh share inspirational information, training, and products that can transform your life.

Ingredients Index

General Index

Numbers

4 by 4 Juice, 198
60-percent solution, 258
80/10/10 Diet, The, 216

A

açai berries, 234
  Berry Best Smoothie, 186
acidosis, 30
acids, balancing, 30-31
acorn squash, Baked Acorn
  Squash, 111
acupuncture, 53-54
agave
  Chia Chocolate Mousse,
   170
  Maca Macaroons, 177
air-filtration systems, 266
alcohol fermentation, 238
alkalines, balancing, 30-31
alkalosis, 30
Almond Miso Soup, 141
Almond Miso Spread/Sauce,
  125
Almond Pad Thai, 168
Almond-Cashew Ice Cream,
  179

almonds
  Almond-Cashew Ice
   Cream, 179
  Almond Miso Soup, 141
  Almond Miso Spread/
   Sauce, 125
  Almond Pad Thai, 168
  Easy Almond Mylk, 95
aloe vera, Berry Best
  Smoothie, 186
aluminum, 17
amino acids, 216-217
anabolic processes, 16
Anderson, Richard, 252
anethole, fennel, 197
anti-aging benefits,
  detoxification, 12-13
anti-inflammatory foods, 12
antibiotics, 33
  overuse, 240
antioxidants, 4, 222-223
Apple Carrot Juice, 196
Apple Ginger Snap Smoothie,
  182
apples
  Apple Carrot Juice, 196
  Apple Ginger Snap, 182
  Avocado Apple Gadget, 157

CAB Juice, 204
Classic Fruit Salad, 158
Collard Wraps, 165
Cucumber Cilantro Juice,
  202
Green Machine Smoothie,
  183
Juice Medley, 200
Apricot Vinaigrette, 135
apricots, Apricot Vinaigrette,
  135
arsenic, 17, 222
asanas (yoga), 48
asbestos, 17
asparagus
  Marinated Veggies, 163
  Nori Rolls, 166
Avocado Apple Gadget, 157
Avocado Dressing, 136
avocados
  Avocado Apple Gadget, 157
  Avocado Dressing, 136
  Creamy Cauliflower
   Sesame Soup, 146
  Garlic Avo Dressing, 134
  Nori Rolls, 166
  Rockin' Guacamole, 153

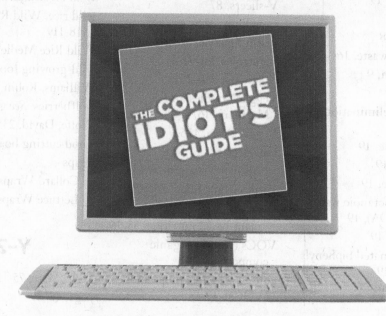